Current Topics in Pathology
91

Managing Editors

C.L. Berry E. Grundmann

Springer
Berlin
Heidelberg
New York
Barcelona
Budapest
Hong Kong
London
Milan
Paris
Santa Clara
Singapore
Tokyo

K.W. Schmid W. Böcker (Eds.)

Thyroid Pathology

Contributors
W. Böcker, J. Brämswig, H. Dralle, R. Gärtner, O. Gimm
H.R. Harach, E. Harms, P.G. Isaacson, B. Jasani, J. Köhrle
D. Ladurner, W. Langsteger, D. Öfner, A. Sakamoto
G.F.W. Scheumann, K.W. Schmid, M. Tötsch
K.-P. Zimmer

Springer

Kurt W. Schmid, Professor Dr.
Werner Böcker, Professor Dr.
University of Münster/Westfalia
Gerhard Domagk Institute of Pathology
Domagkstr. 17
48149 Münster, Germany

With 44 Figures and 20 Tables

ISBN-13: 978-3-642-64446-7 e-ISBN-13: 978-3-642-60531-4
DOI: 10.1007/978-3-642-60531-4

Library of Congress Cataloging-in-Publication Data. Thyroid pathology/K.W. Schmid, W. Bocker, editors. p. cm.—(Current topics in pathology: 91) Includes bibliographical references and index. ISBN-13: 978-3-642-64446-7 1. Thyroid gland—Diseases. 2. Thyroid gland—Pathophysiology. 3. Pathology, Surgical. I. Schmid, Kurt W. II. Bocker, W. (Werner), 1944- . III. Series: Current topics in pathology: v.91. [DNLM: 1. Thyroid Neoplasms—physiopathology. 2. Thyroid Neoplasms—pathology. W1 CU821H v.91 1997/WK 270 T5495 1997] RB1.E6 vol. 91 RC655.49 616.07 s—dc20 [616.4′407] DNLM/DLC for Library of Congress 96-38761

Softcover reprint of the hardcover 1st edition 1997

Cover design: Design & Production GmbH, Heidelberg

Typesetting: Best-set Typesetter Ltd., Hong Kong

SPIN: 10539807 25/3135/SPS - 5 4 3 2 1 0 - Printed on acid-free paper

List of Contributors

Böcker, W., Prof. Dr.	Gerhard Domagk Institute of Pathology University of Münster/Westfalia Domagkstrasse 17 48149 Münster, Germany
Brämswig, J., Prof. Dr.	Pediatric Clinic University of Münster/Westfalia Albert-Schweitzer-Strasse 33 48129 Münster, Germany
Dralle, H., Prof. Dr.	Chirurgische Klinik der Martin-Luther-Universität University of Halle/Saale Magdeburgerstrasse 14 16112 Halle, Germany
Gärtner, R., Prof. Dr.	Medical Clinic Klinikum Innenstadt University of Munich Ziemssenstrasse 1 80336 Munich, Germany
Gimm, O., Dr.	Chirurgische Klinik der Martin-Luther-Universität University of Halle/Saale Magdeburgerstrasse 14 16112 Halle, Germany
Harach, H.R., Dr.	Department of Histopathology Addenbrooke's Hospital Cambridge CB2 2QQ, UK
Harms, E., Prof. Dr.	Pediatric Clinic University of Münster/Westfalia Albert-Schweitzer-Strasse 33 48129 Münster, Germany

ISAACSON, P.G., Prof. Dr.
Department of Histopathology
University College London
Medical School
Rockefeller Building, University Street
London WC1E 6JJ, UK

JASANI, B., Dr.
Immunocytochemistry and Molecular Pathology Unit
Department of Pathology
University of Wales College of Medicine
Cardiff CF4 4XN, UK

KÖHRLE, J., Prof. Dr.
Medical Policlinic
University of Würzburg
Röntgenring 11
97070 Würzburg, Germany

LADURNER, D., Prof. Dr.
Chirurgische Abteilung
Bezirkskrankenhaus St. Johann/Tirol
Austria

LANGSTEGER, W., Univ.-Doz. Dr.
Department of Internal Medicine
Hospital Barmherzige Brüder
Eggenberg
Bergstrasse 27
8021 Graz, Austria

ÖFNER, D., Univ.-Doz. Dr.
Department of Surgery I
University of Innsbruck
Anichstrasse 35
6020 Innsbruck, Austria

SAKAMOTO, A., Prof. Dr.
Department of Pathology
Faculty of Medicine
The University of Tokyo
Hongo, Bunkyo-ku, Tokyo 113, Japan

SCHEUMANN, G.F.W., Dr.
Klinik für Abdominal- und Transplantationschirurgie
University of Hannover
Konstanty-Gutschow-Strasse 8
30625 Hannover, Germany

SCHMID, K.W., Prof. Dr.
Gerhard Domagk Institute of Pathology
University of Münster/Westfalia
48149 Münster, Germany

TÖTSCH, M.,
Univ.-Doz. Dr.

Department of Pathology
University of Innsbruck
Müllerstrasse 44
6020 Innsbruck, Austria

ZIMMER, K.-P.,
Priv.-Doz. Dr.

Pediatric Clinic
University of Münster/Westfalia
Albert-Schweitzer-Strasse 33
48129 Münster, Germany

Preface

Recent years have seen the publication of a number of excellent textbooks dealing with pathology of the thyroid gland. For the present issue of *Current Topics in Pathology* it was thus particularly difficult to select contributions which may offer further information for both pathologists and clinicians. The papers written for this issue can be divided into two sections: The first section addresses the surgical pathology of the thyroid while the second is primarily dedicated to basic aspects of thyroid metabolism, hormone transport, and growth factors in thyroid cells.

The observation of close histological and clinical similarities between low-grade B-cell lymphomas in various organs such as stomach, salivary gland, lung and thyroid has led to the proposal of the MALT (mucosa-associated lymphoid tissue) lymphoma concept. Dr. ISAACSON gives an excellent overview of this notoriously difficult problem in thyroid pathology. Dr. HARACH provides evidence that at least some thyroid C-cell carcinomas may arise from a pluripotent ultimobranchial stem cell. The histopathological diagnosis of both thyroid lymphomas and C-cell carcinomas is based on immunohistochemistry. Dr. JASANI's article deals exclusively with immunohistochemical markers as tools for diagnosis, differentiation and prognosis. Another problem of routine thyroid pathology, namely minimally invasive follicular carcinoma, is addressed in our own contribution (SCHMID and co-workers). Dr. SAKAMOTO describes in his article poorly differentiated carcinoma of the thyroid, a tumour type so far not included in the WHO classification of thyroid tumours. Its morphological and clinical features distinguish this aggressive tumour clearly from both differentiated (follicular and papillary) and anaplastic carcinoma. Dr. GIMM and co-workers emphasise the need for thyroidectomy and lymphadenectomy in papillary thyroid carcinoma.

In the second part, Dr. GÄRTNER describes the mechanisms of various growth factors on thyroid cells. These growth factors apparently mediate both the maintenance of growth and the paracrine communication to fibroblasts and endothelial cells. Dr. KÖHRLE's contribution deals with the key enzyme of thyroid hormone activation, the selenoenzyme type I 5′-deiodinase, the expression of which seems to be closely associated with thyroid differentiation. In an immunoelectronmicroscopical study it is shown by Dr. ZIMMER and co-workers that IgG uptake of thyrocytes in patients suffering from thyroid autoimmune disease from blood circulation takes place at the basolateral membrane; subsequently IgG is transported via a transcytotic pathway to the apical membrane where IgG can be targeted to thyroid autoantigens. Finally, Dr. LANGSTEGER gives a comprehensive overview of the clinical and diagnostic aspects of thyroid hormone transport protein abnormalities.

The contributions in the present issue should be considered as adjuncts to common textbooks on thyroid pathology. We hope in addition that they may help pathologists in their routine diagnostic work as well as stimulate further research in this important field.

Münster, October 1996

KURT W. SCHMID
WERNER BÖCKER

Contents

Lymphoma of the Thyroid Gland

P.G. Isaacson

1 Introduction

Lymphoma of the thyroid is uncommon but its exact incidence is unknown. Thyroid lymphoma almost always arises against a background of Hashimoto's thyroiditis, the relative risk of a patient with Hashimoto's thyroiditis developing lymphoma being 67 (Holm et al. 1985). In 1984 Isaacson and Wright noted close histological and clinical similarities between low- grade B-cell lymphomas of the stomach, salivary gland, lung and thyroid. The histological features of these lymphomas appeared to recapitulate those of mucosa-associated lymphoid tissue (MALT), as typified by Peyer's patches, and the term "MALT lymphoma" was coined to describe this group of extranodal lymphomas (Isaacson and Wright 1984). Unlike the other common sites where MALT lymphomas occur, the thyroid cannot be described as a mucosal organ. As the MALT concept has developed, however, it has become clear that the common theme is not necessarily that the lymphomas arise in mucosae but, rather, that they arise from acquired lymphoid tissue with features of MALT; these include lymphoid follicles and adjacent epithelium containing intraepithelial B-cells, the so-called lymphoepithelium. Functionally, MALT differs from nodal lymphoid tissue in that antigens gain access directly across the lymphoepithelium rather than via afferent lymphatics.

MALT lymphomas tend to arise in a setting of those autoimmune diseases which are characterized by acquisition of MALT. The lymphomas share common histological features which may be difficult to differentiate from those of the lymphoid infiltrate which characterizes the preceding autoimmune disorder itself

Current Topics in Pathology
Volume 91, K.W. Schmid/W. Böcker (Eds.)

without resorting to special techniques to demonstrate monoclonality. The clinical course of low-grade MALT lymphomas is characterized by a tendency to remain localized, and dissemination, when it occurs, is to "mucosal" sites, with sparing of the bone marrow. Transformation to high-grade lymphoma can occur.

Despite the biological and clinical homogeneity of low-grade B-cell thyroid lymphomas, pathologists have continued to apply a wide variety of terms to them, implying that a group of different tumours [e.g. follicular (CB/CC) lymphoma, diffuse small cleaved (mantle cell) lymphoma, lymphocytic lymphoma (CLL), monocytoid B-cell lymphoma and plasmacytoma] arise in a common background of Hashimoto's thyroiditis (Aozasa 1986a,b, 1987; Mizukami et al. 1990). In the light of the MALT concept it becomes clear that these "different" thyroid lymphomas are, in fact, a single clinicopathological lymphoma variant, namely low- or high-grade MALT-type lymphoma.

2 Thyroid Lymphoid Tissue

In common with other sites where MALT lymphomas arise, the thyroid gland contains no native lymphoid tissue. Lymphoid tissue acquired in the course of Hashimoto's thyroiditis, like that acquired by the salivary gland in Sjögren's syndrome (Hyjek et al. 1988), bears a close resemblance to MALT (Hyjek and Isaacson 1988); it is characterized by the presence of B-cell follicles, infiltration of thyroid epithelium by B cells (the so-called lymphoepithelium), and plasma cell differentiation (Fig. 1). Because the thyroid is an endocrine gland without ducts, the histological resemblance to Peyer's patches, which characterizes acquired MALT in the salivary gland and other mucosal organs, is more subtle. In comparison with acquired MALT in other sites, plasma cell differentiation is much more marked.

The borderline between low-grade B-cell MALT lymphoma of the thyroid and its benign reactive precursor, Hashimoto's thyroiditis, can be difficult to define on morphological grounds alone. The remarkably indolent clinical behaviour characteristic of low-grade thyroid MALT lymphoma serves to accentuate this difficulty and underlines the relationship between the two lesions. This was well illustrated by Hyjek and Isaacson (1988), who, following a careful analysis of thyroid glands from 236 patients treated surgically for Hashimoto's thyroiditis, identified five unsuspected low-grade MALT lymphomas.

3 Thyroid Lymphoma of MALT Type

3.1 Clinical Presentation

Most thyroid lymphomas, like Hashimoto's disease, occur in females over 50 years old. Recurrent thyroid enlargement in a patient with a goitre and/or stable

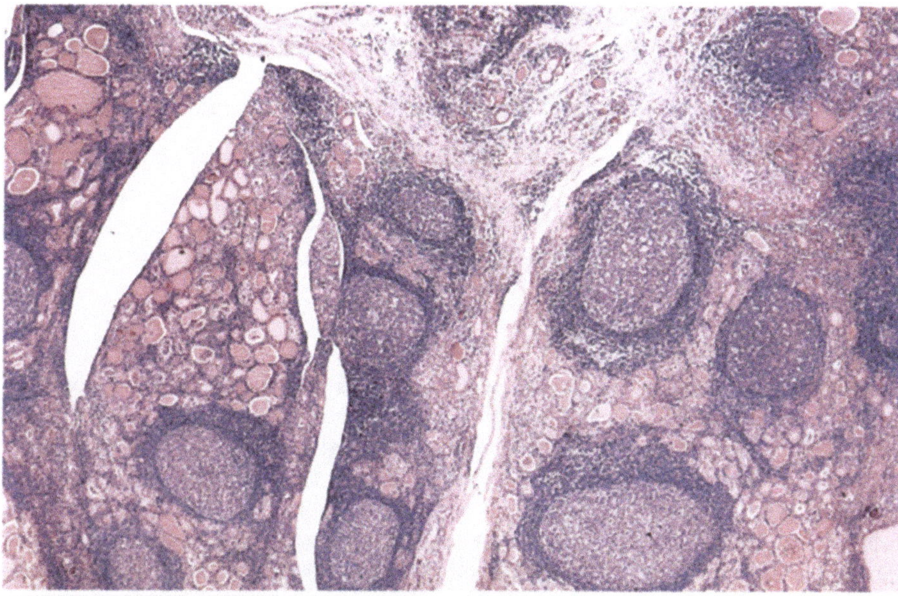

a

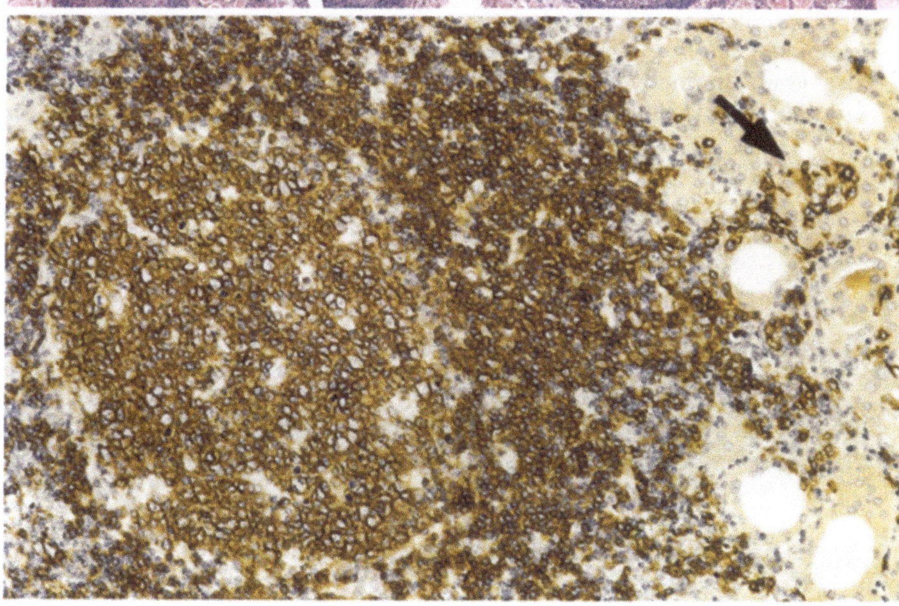

b

Fig. 1. a Hashimoto's thyroiditis showing prominent B-cell follicles. **b** Same case at higher magnification, immunostained with CD20 to show B cells extending into adjacent thyroid acinar epithelium (*arrow*)

Hashimoto's thyroiditis is a characteristic. There may be no documented history of Hashimoto's thyroiditis, but serology will usually reveal the presence of thyroid auto-antibodies. Rapid growth of the thyroid, dysphagia and hoarseness are symptoms more suggestive of poorly differentiated carcinoma but may herald the onset of high-grade lymphoma.

3.2 Histopathology

3.2.1 Low-Grade MALT Lymphoma

In the thyroid, high- rather than low-grade B-cell lymphoma is more common in most published series, but whether this is truly representative of thyroid lymphoma is uncertain. In some high-grade cases a low-grade component is present, but just how often this occurs is unclear since a careful search - not always possible in archival material - may be necessary to reveal the low-grade component. Thus, as is the case in other MALT lymphomas (Chan et al. 1990), at least some and possibly most high-grade cases are the result of evolution of low-grade lymphoma that may have been present for many years but remained undiagnosed.

Low-grade thyroid lymphoma characteristically occurs against a background of Hashimoto's thyroiditis as either focal or diffuse areas of confluent, dense

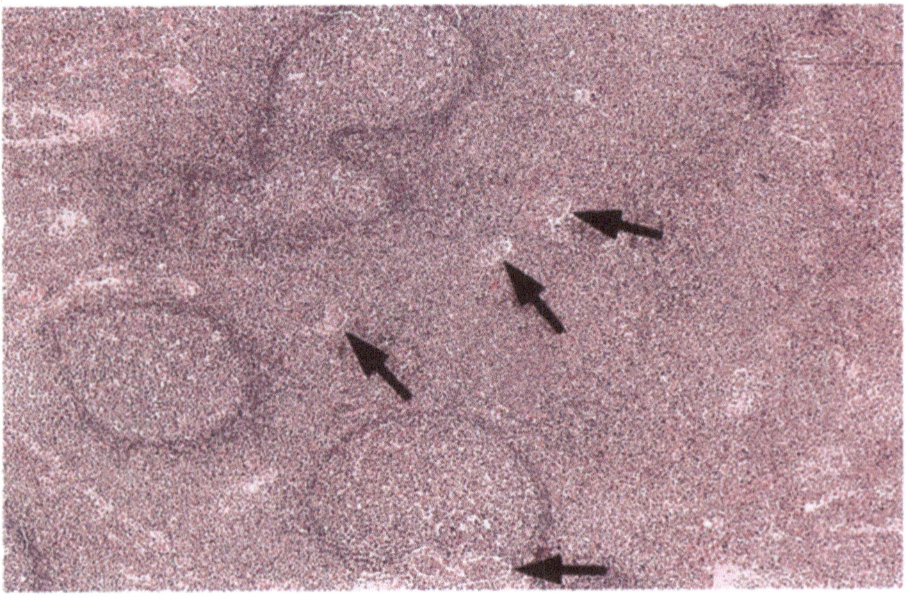

Fig. 2. Low-grade B-cell MALT lymphoma of thyroid showing diffuse infiltration of thyroid with scattered residual B-cell follicles. Lymphoepithelial lesions can just be seen (*arrows*)

lymphoid infiltration with effacement of thyroid acini (HYJEK and ISAACSON 1988) (Fig. 2). Reactive lymphoid follicles are always present and may be extremely prominent. The lymphomatous infiltrate is centred around the follicles, displacing surviving thyroid tissue peripherally; this appearance is better appreciated in immunohistochemically stained preparations (see below). The lymphomatous infiltrate is characteristic of low-grade MALT lymphoma, consisting of centrocyte-like (CCL) cells which form lymphoepithelial lesions with thyroid acini (Fig. 3). These lymphoepithelial lesions are often very prominent even at low power (Fig. 2). The cytological features of the CCL cells show the characteristic range of appearances, resembling either small lymphocytes, centrocytes or monocytoid B cells (Figs. 4–6). Scattered transformed blasts are nearly always present. In comparison with other MALT lymphomas, plasma cell differentiation is more prominent in thyroid lymphoma (Fig. 7). It may be so extreme as to suggest a diagnosis of plasmacytoma and many cases have indeed been diagnosed as such; in these cases the characteristic CCL cells are most easily identified in and around lymphoepithelial lesions which are not formed by the non-invasive plasma cells but by CCL B cells (Fig. 7). Immunohistochemistry can be helpful in this respect (see below).

Colonization of the reactive B-cell follicles by the neoplastic CCL cells has been well described in thyroid MALT lymphoma (ISAACSON et al. 1992). This follicular colonization can take three forms. The most frequent pattern is for reactive follicles to be colonized by CCL cells; this can lead to a resemblance, often marked, to

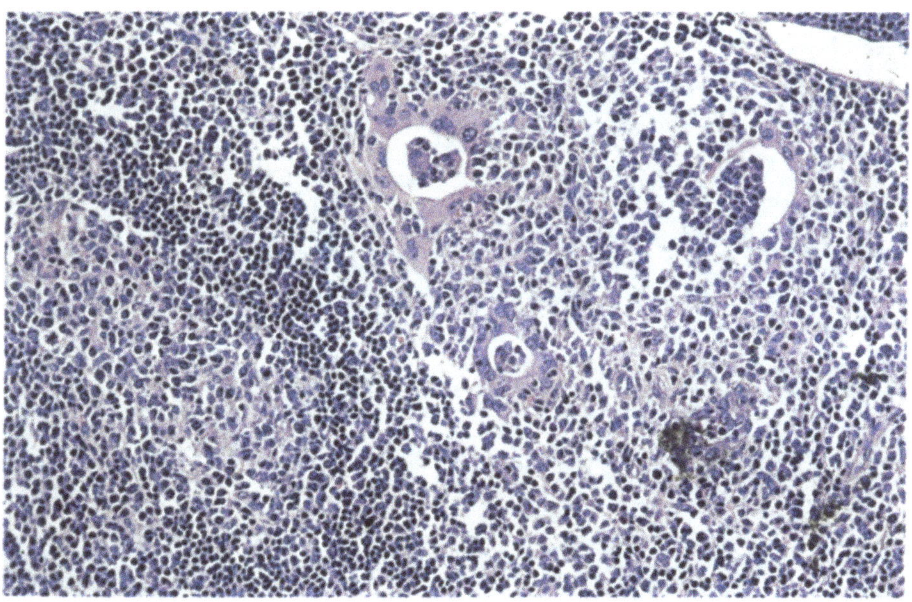

Fig. 3. Low-grade B-cell lymphoma of thyroid showing the characteristic features of MALT lymphoma, with a follicle (*left*) adjacent to which are centrocyte-like cells which infiltrate thyroid acini forming lymphoepithelial lesions

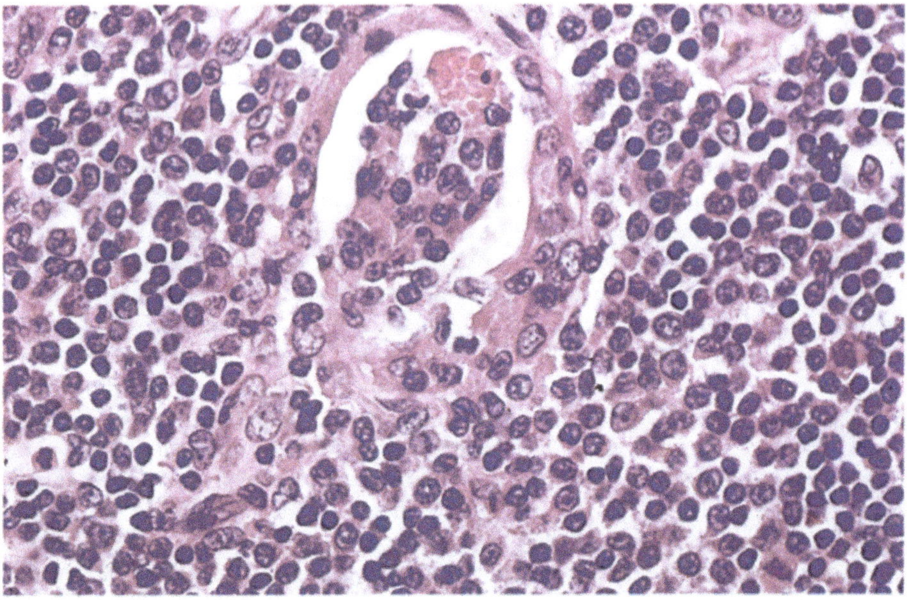

Fig. 4. Cytological section of low-grade B-cell MALT lymphoma in which the cells resemble small lymphocytes. Note the lymphoepithelial lesion

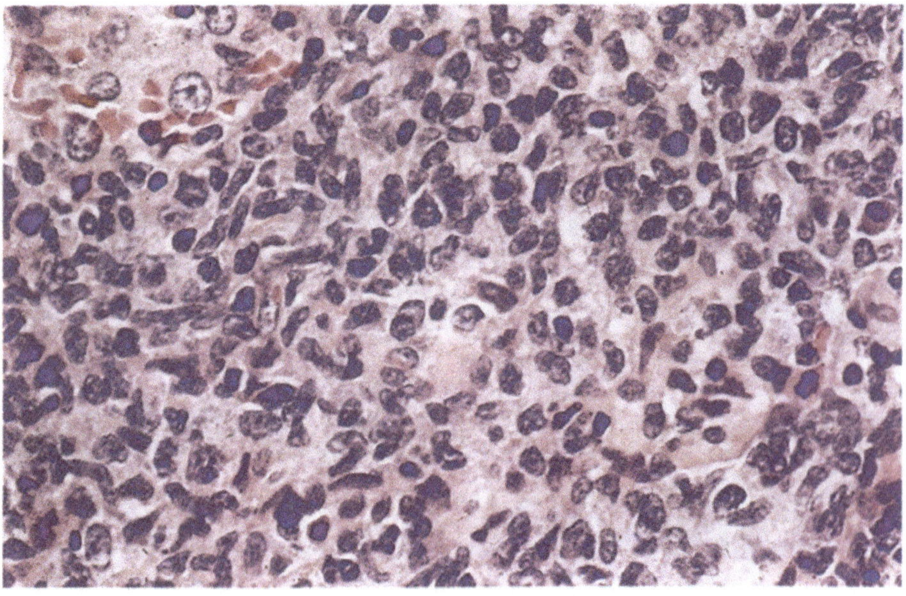

Fig. 5. In this low-grade B-cell MALT lymphoma of the thyroid the cells are centrocyte-like

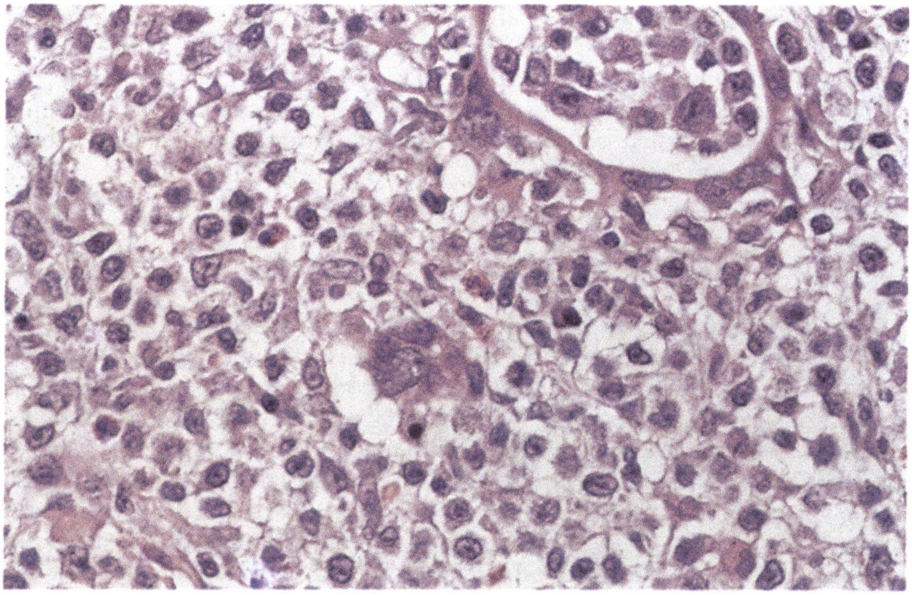

Fig. 6. The cells in this low-grade B-cell MALT lymphoma of the thyroid have a monocytoid appearance

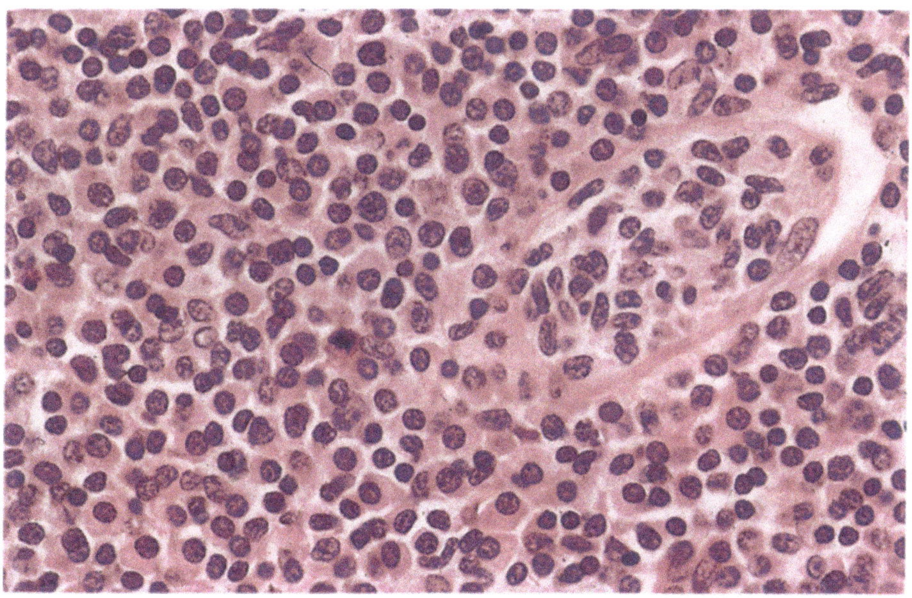

Fig. 7. Plasma cell differentiation in low-grade B-cell MALT lymphoma of the thyroid; a lymphoepithelial lesion is present on the *right*

follicular (CB/CC) lymphoma (Fig. 8). Usually, the cells within the follicle centres, become slightly enlarged and show greater numbers of mitotic figures in comparison to the diffuse interfollicular infiltrate. Less commonly, the cells within colonized follicles are unchanged in comparison to those comprising the diffuse infiltrate or show plasma cell differentiation which can only be detected using immunohistochemistry (see below).

3.2.2 High-Grade B-Cell Lymphoma

High-grade transformation of low-grade MALT lymphoma may occur focally (Fig. 9); alternatively, most or all sections of the thyroid may show a high-grade tumour. In either case the histological and cytological appearances of the high-grade lymphoma are similar. Sheets of tumour cells replace the thyroid and neither reactive follicles nor plasma cell differentiation are present. Unlike in other high-grade MALT lymphomas, lymphoepithelial lesions can often be found (Bateman and Wright 1993). Any surviving thyroid usually shows evidence of Hashimoto's disease. Cytologically, the high-grade lymphoma cells are not distinctive; they may resemble centroblasts or immunoblasts or show the features of neither.

3.3 Immunohistochemistry

Unlike other MALT lymphomas, in which the tumour cells with few exceptions synthesize IgM, the predominant immunoglobulin in thyroid MALT lymphoma is

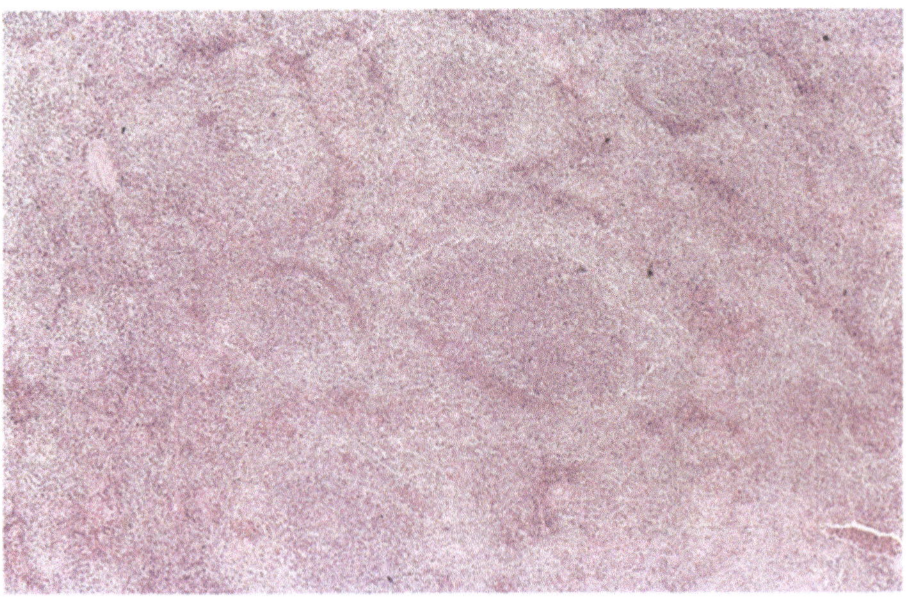

Fig. 8. Follicular colonization in low-grade B-cell MALT lymphoma of thyroid

a

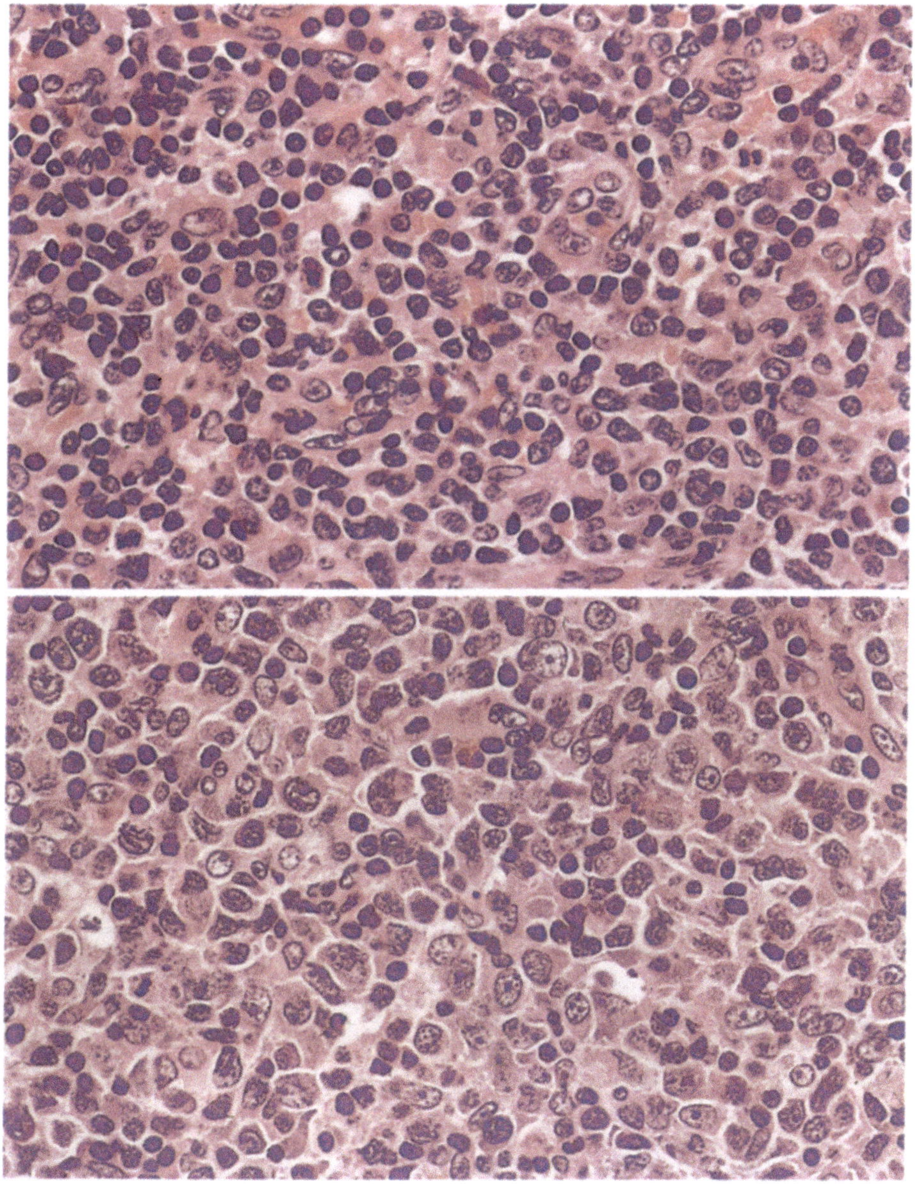

b

Fig. 9. **a** Low-grade B-cell MALT lymphoma of the thyroid showing **b** high-grade transformation

IgG. Because of the usually marked degree of plasma cell differentiation, low-grade thyroid MALT lymphomas light chain restriction can usually be easily demonstrated in paraffin sections (Fig. 10). In those cases in which plasma cells predominate, staining with CD20 is useful to demonstrate the B-cell component and

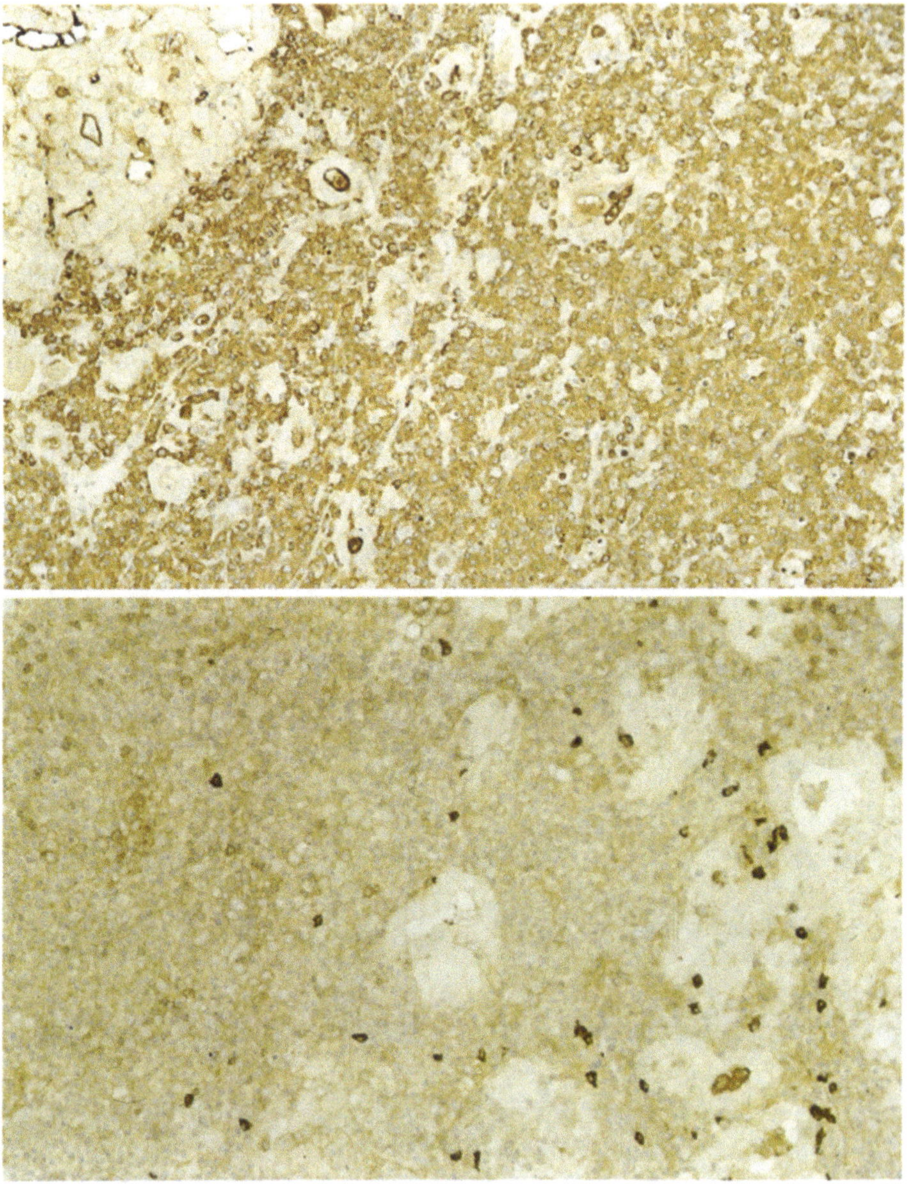

a

b

Fig. 10a,b. Low-grade thyroid MALT lymphoma with marked plasma cell differentiation stained **a** for κ immunoglobulin light chain and **b** for λ light chain. There is κ light chain restriction

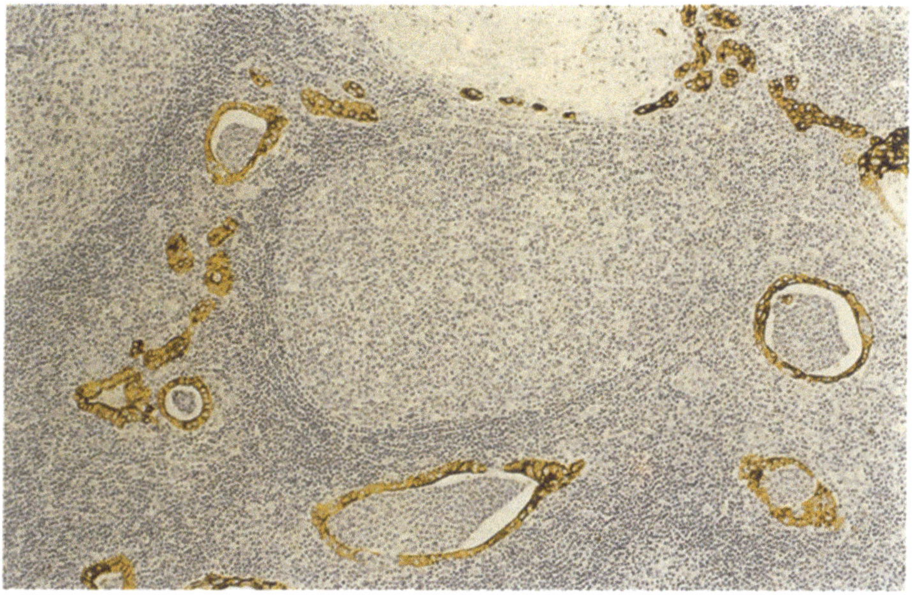

Fig. 11. Low-grade B-cell MALT lymphoma of the thyroid stained for cytokeratin, which highlights the perifollicular distribution and lymphoepithelial lesions

lymphoepithelial lesions. Lymphoepithelial lesions are also well shown with antibodies to cytokeratin, which also highlight the perifollicular pattern of the lymphomatous infiltrate (Fig. 11).

The reactive B-cell follicles normally show polytypic staining with antibodies to immunoglobulin light chains, but in cases showing follicular colonization CCL or plasma cells in the follicle centres show immunoglobulin light chain restriction (Fig. 12). Colonized follicles associated with "activation" of CCL cells show loss of reactivity with antibodies to *bcl-2* protein in contrast to true follicular (CB/CC) lymphoma, and the proliferation fraction of the intrafollicular tumour cells is greatly increased in contrast to the interfollicular infiltrate (Fig. 13).

3.4 Molecular Genetics

The presence of clonal immunoglobulin gene rearrangement distinguishes low-grade MALT lymphoma from florid Hashimoto's disease. In common with other MALT lymphomas, thyroid lymphomas, including those with a spurious follicular pattern, do not show *bcl-2* gene rearrangement (Isaacson et al. 1992).

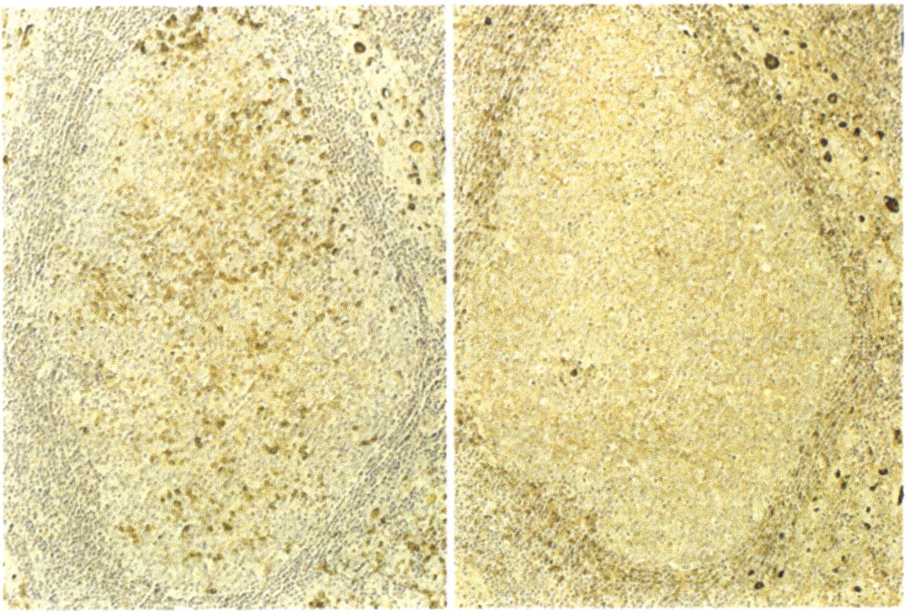

a b

Fig. 12a,b. Thyroid MALT lymphoma stained **a** for κ immunoglobulin light chain and **b** for λ light chain. Plasma cells within a reactive follicle centre show κ light chain restriction

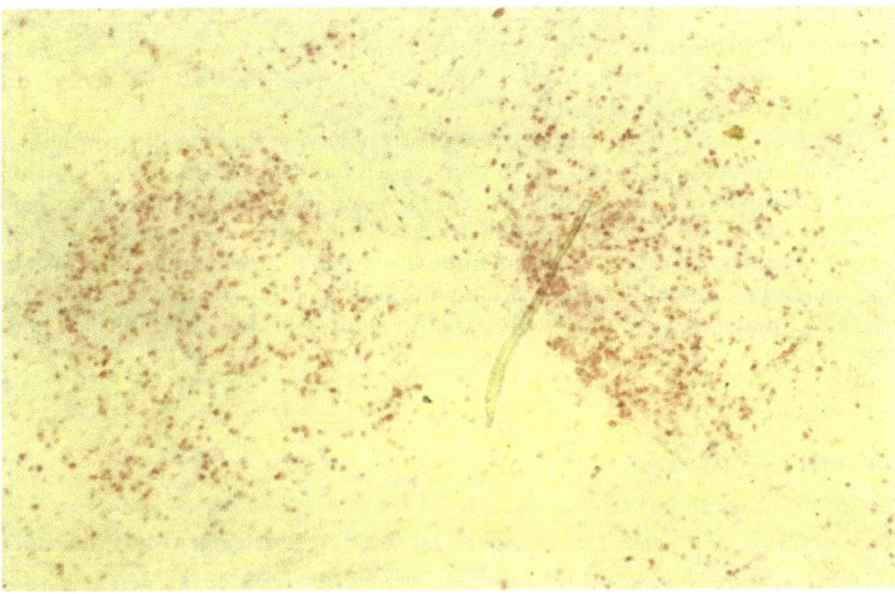

Fig. 13. Follicular colonization in low-grade B-cell MALT lymphoma of thyroid stained with Ki67, showing a high proliferation fraction of the cells which have colonized follicle centres compared to the interfollicular infiltrate

3.5 Differential Diagnosis

With the advent of immunohistochemistry the distinction between either low- or high-grade lymphoma and small- or large-cell thyroid carcinoma no longer poses a problem. Rarely, the thyroid may be the principal, or, even more rarely, the primary focus of true follicular (CB/CC) lymphoma. By contrast with thyroid MALT lymphomas showing follicular colonization, follicular lymphomas do not form lymphoepithelial lesions or show plasma cell differentiation, and the uninvolved thyroid gland does not, except by chance, show Hashimoto's disease. Immunohistochemistry will distinguish CD10-positive, *bcl-2* protein-positive, follicular lymphoma from MALT lymphoma with follicular colonization, which usually shows a reciprocal staining profile. By contrast with follicular lymphoma, *bcl-2* gene rearrangement is not present in thyroid MALT lymphoma (Isaacson et al. 1992). Lymphocytic lymphoma (CLL) may involve the thyroid. In these rare cases neither reactive follicles, plasma cell differentiation nor lymphoepithelial lesions are a feature, and this lymphoma is typically CD5-positive.

3.6 Clinical Behaviour

There are no really adequate follow-up studies in patients with low-grade MALT lymphoma of the thyroid, but prolonged disease-free survival following thyroidectomy has been documented (Hyjek and Isaacson 1988; Anscombe and Wright 1985; Compagno and Oertel 1980). Those cases of high-grade thyroid lymphoma confined by the capsule of the gland (stage I_E) have a good prognosis even in the presence of lymph node involvement (stage II_E). Capsular invasion, however, results in a much poorer prognosis similar to that of stage III and IV nodal lymphoma (Burke et al. 1977). Primary thyroid lymphomas have a tendency to disseminate to the gastrointestinal tract (McDermott et al. 1992). In the case of low-grade lymphomas, the gastrointestinal secondary may recapitulate the features of MALT lymphoma, including the formation of lymphoepithelial lesions.

References

Anscombe AM, Wright DH (1985) Primary malignant lymphoma of the thyroid – a tumour of mucosa-associated lymphoid tissue: review of seventy-six cases. Histopathology 9: 81–97

Aozasa K, Inoue A, Yoshimura H et al (1986a) Plasmacytoma of the thyroid gland. Cancer 58: 105–110

Aozasa K, Inoue A, Yoshimura H et al (1986b) Intermediate lymphocytic lymphoma of the thyroid. An immunologic and immunohistologic study. Cancer 57: 1762–1767

Aozasa K, Ueda T, Katagiri S et al (1987) Immunologic and immunohistologic analysis of 27 cases with thyroid lymphomas. Cancer 60: 969–973

Bateman AC, Wright DH (1993) High-grade MALT lymphomas of the thyroid show epitheliotropism. J Pathol 169 Suppl 142A

Burke JS, Butler JJ, Fuller LM (1977) Malignant lymphomas of the thyroid: a clinical pathologic study of 35 patients including ultrastructural observations. Cancer 39: 1587–1602

Chan JKC, Ng CS, Isaacson PG (1990) Relationship between high-grade lymphoma and low-grade B-cell mucosa-associated lymphoid tissue lymphoma (MALToma) of the stomach. Am J Pathol 13: 1023–1033

Compagno J, Oertel JE (1980) Malignant lymphoma and other lymphoproliferative disorders of the thyroid gland. A clinicopathologic study of 245 cases. Am J Clin Pathol 74: 1–11

Holm L-E, Blomgren H, Löwhagen T (1985) Cancer risks in patients with chronic lymphocytic thyroidits. N Engl J Med 312: 601–604

Hyjek E, Isaacson PG (1988) Primary B cell lymphoma of the thyroid and its relationship to Hashimoto's thyroiditis. Hum Pathol 19: 1315–1326

Hyjek E, Smith WJ, Isaacson PG (1988) Primary B-cell lymphoma of salivary glands and its relationship to myoepithelial sialadenitis. Hum Pathol 19: 766–776

Isaacson PG, Wright DH (1984) Extranodal malignant lymphoma arising from mucosa-associated lymphoid tissue. Cancer 53: 2515–2524

Isaacson PG, Androulakis-Papachristou A, Diss TC et al (1992) Follicular colonization in thyroid lymphoma. Am J Pathol 141: 43–52

McDermott EWM, Cassidy N, Heffernan SJ (1992) Perforation through undiagnosed small bowel involvement in primary thyroid lymphoma during chemotherapy. Cancer 69: 572–573

Mizukami Y, Michigishi T, Nonomura A et al (1990) Primary lymphoma of the thyroid: a clinical, histological and immunohistochemical study of 20 cases. Histopathology 17: 201–209

Histogenesis of Thyroid C-Cell Carcinoma

H.R. HARACH

The origin of medullary carcinoma of the thyroid (MCT) from the "parafollicular cells" was recognised by WILLIAMS in 1966, seven years after its identification as a distinct clinico-pathological entity by HAZARD et al. (1959). In contrast to tumours of follicular cell origin, which produce thyroid hormones and thyroglobulin (KAWAOI et al. 1982), the neoplastic C cells synthesize the calcium-lowering hormone calcitonin (MILHAUD et al. 1965). Their differences are further highlighted by epidemiological data. Radiation, high iodine intake and race are related particularly to papillary carcinoma, whilst low iodine intake, as seen in goitrous areas, and dyshormonogenesis, ore more related to follicular carcinoma (WILLIAMS 1979). MCT has been described to occur after prolonged hypercalcaemia (LIVOLSI and FEIND 1979). Experimental studies would also support a major role of dietary calcium and vitamin D for the generation of C-cell tumours (WILLIAMS 1979). MCT is inherited in about 20% of the cases as an autosomal dominant trait (WILLIAMS 1979) linked to the pericentromeric region of chromosome 10 which shows *ret* point mutations as often do sporadic MCTs (MULLIGAN and PONDER 1995). Inherited MCT is usually accompanied or preceded by C-cell hyperplasia (DELELLIS and WOLFE 1981), which would further support its C-cell origin.

The existence of a second type of epithelial cell or "parenchymatous cells" in the thyroid was suggested in 1876 by BABER on the basis of studies in the dog. GETZOWA in 1907 and GODWIN in 1937 suggested that these cells derived from the ultimobranchial contribution to the thyroid, whilst NONIDEZ in 1932 used silver impregnation to separate "parafollicular cells" from follicular cells. The term "C cell" was introduced by PEARSE in 1966 due to their calcitonin content, and parafollicular cells have been identified in developing human ultimobranchial body (CHAN and CONEN 1971). The work of LE DOUARIN and LE LIEVRE in 1970, however, showed, using quail chick transplant experiments, that C cells are derived from the neural crest. The production of nerve growth factor by MCT (CRAMER et al. 1979) would support this concept, but further evidence for and against these findings remains. The genetic association of MCT with neurinomata and phaeochromocytoma in MEN2b would semantically support the neural crest origin of C cells, but neither MEN2a, which is often associated with parathyroid disease (WILLIAMS 1967), nor the existence of mixed medullary-follicular tumours in the context of familial MCT would do so (MIZUKAMI et al. 1993; NOEL et al. 1991). Melanocytic cells have been described in occasional MCT (MARCUS et al. 1982), and human neoplastic C cells in culture may elicit action potentials (TISCHLER et al. 1976). These two phenomena have also been observed in phaeochromocytoma and in tumours of the diffuse endocrine system (CHETTY et

Current Topics in Pathology
Volume 91, K.W. Schmid/W. Böcker (Eds.)

al. 1993; Grazer et al. 1982; Tischler et al. 1976), the latter now largely not thought to be neural crest-derivative tissue (Andrew 1982; Wright 1990). MCT and normal C cells may produce several hormonal polypeptides and so-called "neuroendocrine markers" (Caillou et al. 1983; Kendall et al. 1986; Lloyd et al. 1983; Schröder et al. 1988; Harach et al. 1992; Schmid et al. 1992), which may also occur in non-endocrine tumours (Wright 1990).

Studies on classic MCTs revealed the presence of neoplastic microfollicles only discernible at electron microscopy and intraluminal glycoproteins (Sobrinho-Simoes et al. 1990). One such glycoprotein had been earlier identified as a high molecular weight thyroglobulin so-called "C thyroglobulin" (Kameda et al. 1979), which is also present in canine C cell complexes (Kameda et al. 1980). This led some authors to consider MCT as a basically glandular tumour (Sobrinho-Simoes et al. 1990); MCTs with obvious glandular components do occur (Harach and Williams 1983). In addition, MCTs showing a variety of neoplastic cells with endodermal differentiation have been described, including mucinous cells (Fernandes et al. 1982; Caillou et al. 1983) and squamous or epidermoid cells (Caillou et al. 1983; Schröder et al. 1988). It appears that the more endodermal-derivative components are searched for in MCT, the lower the frequency of pure C-cell carcinomas the pathologist will be left with. Indeed, up to 58% of MCTs were found to produce mucin (Martin-Lacave et al. 1988), whereas follicles with acid mucin lined by abundant C cells occasionally showing intracytoplasmic mucus have been described in the normal human thyroid (Harach 1985a). MCT shows cytokeratin immunoreaction (Schröder et al. 1988), whilst carcinoembryonic antigen, a preferentially gut-associated marker, is also expressed by normal and neoplastic C cells (Lloyd et al. 1983; Schröder et al. 1988).

The observations of tumours showing a C-cell component together with follicular cells (e.g. mixed medullary-follicular carcinoma) (Hales et al. 1982) have, again, given rise to speculation as to whether at least some human C cells are of endodermal origin (Harach 1985a, 1991), comparable to the derivation of endocrine cells found in the gut (Wright 1990). Ultimobranchial cysts in human subjects with undescended thyroid glands were found to contain both follicular and C cells (Williams et al. 1989), which are also present in the human ultimobranchially related thyroid follicles with acid mucin (Harach 1985a, 1991). This adds support to the belief that some follicular cells originate in the lateral thyroid anlagen (Williams et al. 1989). Further support to the dual cell origin concept is given by the description of occasional mixed medullary-follicular carcinomas in patients with familial antecedents of MCT (Mizukami et al. 1993; Noel et al. 1991). Not least, human mixed follicular-parafollicular cell tumours were found to show similar morphological and histochemical features to ultimobranchial tumours in bulls (Ljungberg and Nilsson 1991).

Mucoepidermoid carcinoma of the thyroid may show a minor C-cell component (Franssila et al. 1984; Sambade et al. 1990). An endodermal ultimobranchial origin has been suggested for this tumour based on its morphological, histochemical, immunohistochemical and ultrastructural resemblance to human fetal (Harach et al. 1993) and postnatal ultimobranchial nests (Harach 1985b,c; Harach and Wasenius 1987). These remnants are mainly composed of non-keratinizing epidermoid cells and mucinous cells, and may contain mucinous material (HARACH 1985b; HARACH et al. 1993) as well as occasional C cells (JANZER et al. 1979; HARACH et al. 1993). They are centrally located in the middle to the upper third of the lateral thyroid lobes (HARACH 1985d; HARACH et al. 1993), as are the C cells (DELELLIS and WOLFE 1981), which are more abundant in thyroid parenchyma close to the ultimobranchial nests (JANZER et al. 1979; HARACH et al. 1993). More recently, thyroglobulin-immunoreactive cells have been described to occur in thyroid mucoepidermoid carcinoma (SAMBADE et al. 1990), as earlier demonstrated in the ultimobranchial solid cell nests and in follicular cells from the so-called mixed follicles (HARACH 1985d). The latter, which are lined by follicular cells on one side and ultimobranchial epidermoid cells on the other, also contain intraluminal mucin (HARACH 1987).

If MCT was derived from neural crest cells, tumours showing features of MCT should have been recognised in proliferations of neurocrest-derived cells (i.e. phaeochromocytoma and paraganglioma). Apart from the presence of occasional calcitonin-immunoreactive cells in a few cases, this has not occurred (CAPELLA et al. 1988). Calcitonin immunoreaction occurs in islet cell and other tumours of the diffuse endocrine system (KLÖPPEL and HEITZ 1988; CHEJFEC et al. 1988) considered to be derived from endoderm (ANDREW 1982; WRIGHT 1990). Furthermore, phaeochromocytes may give rise to phaeochromocytomas, occasionally combined with other neurocrest-derived neoplastic tissue components such as ganglioneuroma (KRAGEL and JOHNSTON 1985) or peripheral nerve sheath tumour (MIN et al. 1988). This has not been reported in MCT which, in contrast, not infrequently shows differentiation towards endodermal derivatives (see above) not yet reported to occur in phaeochromocytoma. Based on all these observations, the possibility that some pure C-cell MCTs originate from a pluripotent ultimobranchial stem cell differentiating towards a restricted C-cell lineage could not be excluded. The temptation to suggest the same hypothesis for some thyroid pure follicular cell proliferations cannot be avoided. Follicular cells in the wall of occasional branchial cysts (PARHAM 1988; DOI et al. 1988) and a laterally situated follicular tumour from a patient with a normally descended thyroid gland (STANTON and ALLEN-MERSH 1984) have been described. By analogy, cleft-like cysts lined by respiratory and squamous epithelia, as found in ultimobranchial cysts (WILLIAMS et al. 1989), may occur in the thyroid (DELABIE et al. 1990). Hopefully, future studies using specific "ultimobranchial tissue markers", molecular biological techniques and experimental models will help to unravel some of the remaining mysteries of this fascinating topic.

Acknowledgement. I wish to thank Professor Sir Dillwyn Williams for his continuous encouragement and suggestions throughout the production of the manuscript.

References

Andrew A (1982) The APUD concept: where has it led us? Br Med Bull 38: 221–225
Baber EC (1876) Contributions to the minute anatomy of the thyroid gland of the dog. Proc R Soc Lond [Biol] 24: 240–241

Caillou B, Talbot M, Schlumberger M, Rougier P, Bellet D, Travagli JP (1983) Usefulness of new methodological and conceptual approaches in thyroid carcinoma (especially in medullary carcinoma). Acta Endocrinol (Copenh) 102 Suppl 252: 29–31
Capella C, Riva C, Cornaggia M, Chiaravalli AM, Frigerio B (1988) Histopathology, cytology and cytochemistry of pheochromocytomas and paragangliomas including chemodectomas. Pathol Res Pract 183: 176–187
Chan AS, Conen PE (1971) Ultrastructural observations on cytodifferentiation of parafollicular cells in the human fetal thyroid. Lab Invest 25: 249–259
Chejfec G, Falkmer S, Askensten U, Grimelius L, Gould VE (1988) Neuroendocrine tumors of the gastrointestinal tract. Pathol Res Pract 183: 143–154
Chetty R, Clark SP, Taylor DA (1993) Pigmented pheochromocytomas of the adrenal medulla. Hum Pathol 24: 420–423
Cramer SF, Bradshaw RA, Balgan NC, Meyers JA (1979) Nerve growth factor in medullary carcinoma of the thyroid. Hum Pathol 10: 731–736
Delabie J, de Wolf-Peeters C, Cappelle L, van Damme B, Desmet V (1990) Branchial cleftlike cysts of the thyroid. Am J Surg Pathol 14: 1165–1166
DeLellis RH, Wolfe HJ (1981) The pathobiology of the human calcitonin (C)-cell: a review. Pathol Annu 2: 25–52
Doi O, Hutson JM, Myers NA, McKelvie PA (1988) Branchial remnants: a review of 58 cases. J Pediatr Surg 23: 789–792
Fernandes BJ, Bedard YC, Rosen I (1982) Mucus-producing medullary cell carcinoma of the thyroid gland. Am J Clin Pathol 78: 536–540
Franssila KO, Harach HR, Wasenius VM (1984) Mucoepidermoid carcinoma of the thyroid. Histopathology 8: 847–860
Getzowa S (1907) Über die Glandula parathyroidea, intrathyroideale Zell-haufen derselben und Reste des postbranchialen Körpers. Virchows Arch [Pathol Anat] 188: 181–234
Godwin MC (1937) Complex IV in the dog with specil emphasis on the relation of the ultimobranchial body to interfollicular cells in the post natal thyroid gland. Am J Anat 60: 299–339
Grazer R, Cohen SM, Jacobs JB, Lucas P (1982) Melanin-containing peripheral carcinoid of the lung. Am J Surg Pathol 6: 73–78
Hales M, Rosenau W, Okerlund MD, Galante M (1982) Carcinoma of the thyroid with a mixed medullary and follicular pattern. Morphologic, immunohistochemical, and clinical laboratory studies. Cancer 50: 1352–1359
Harach HR (1985a) Thyroid follicles with acid mucin in man. A second kind of follicles? Cell Tissus Res 242: 211–215
Harach HR (1985b) A study on the relationship between solid cell nests and mucoepidermoid carcinoma of the thyroid. Histopathology 9: 195–207
Harach HR (1985c) Histological markers of solid cell nests of the thyroid. With some emphasis on their expression in thyroid ultimobranchial-related tumors. Acta Anat (Basel) 124: 111–116
Harach HR (1985d) Solid cell nests of the thyroid. An anatomical survey and immunohistochemical study for the presence of thyroglobulin. Acta Anat (Basel) 122: 249–253
Harach HR (1987) Mixed follicles of the human thyroid. Acta Anat (Basel) 129: 27–30
Harach HR (1991) Thyroglobulin in human thyroid follicles with acid mucin. J Pathol 164: 261–263
Harach HR, Wasenius VM (1987) Expression of "visceral" cytokeratin and ultrastructural findings in solid cell nests of the thyroid. Acta Anat (Basel) 129: 289–292
Harach HR, Williams ED (1983) Glandular (tubular and follicular) variants of medullary carcinoma of the thyroid. Histopathology 7: 83–97
Harach HR, Wilander E, Grimelius L, Bergholm U, Westermark P, Falkmer S (1992) Chromogranin A immunoreactivity compared with argyrophilia, calcitonin immunoreactivity, and amyloid as tumour markers in the histopathological diagnosis of medullary (C-cell) carcinoma. Pathol Res Pract 188: 123–130
Harach HR, Vujanic GM, Jasani B (1993) Ultimobranchial body nests in human fetal thyroid: an autopsy, histological, and immunohistochemical study in relation to solid cell nests and mucoepidermoid carcinoma of the thyroid. J Pathol 169: 465–469

Hazard JB, Hawk WA, Crile G Jr (1959) Medullary (solid) carcinoma of the thyroid: a clinicopathologic entity. J Clin Endocrinol Metab 19: 152–161
Janzer RC, Weber E, Hedinger C (1979) The relation between solid cell nests and C cells of the thyroid gland. Cell Tissue Res 197: 295–312
Kameda Y, Harada T, Ito K, Ikeda A (1979) Immunohistochemical study of the medullary thyroid carcinoma with reference to C-thyroglobulin reaction of tumor cells. Cancer 44: 2071–2082
Kameda Y, Shigemoto H, Ikeda A (1980) Development and cytodifferentiation of C cell complexes in dog feltal thyroids. An immunohistochemical study using anti-calcitonin, anti-C thyroglobulin and anti 19S thyroglobulin antisera. Cell Tissue Res 206: 403–415
Kawaoi A, Okano T, Nemoto N, Shiina Y, Shikata T (1982) Simultaneous detection of thyroglobulin (Tg), thyroxine (T4), and triiodothyronine (T3) in nontoxic thyroid tumors by the immunoperoxidase method. Am J Pathol 108: 39–49
Kendall CH, Homer CE, Bishop AE, Polak JM (1986) Age-related peptide production by human thyroid C cells. An immunohistochemical study. Virchows Arch [A] 410: 97–101
Klöppel G, Heitz PU (1988) Pancreatic endocrine tumors. Pathol Res Pract 183: 155–168
Kragel PJ, Johnston CA (1985) Pheochromocytoma-ganglioneuroma of the adrenal. Arch Pathol Lab Med 109: 470–472
Le Douarin N, Le Lievre C (1970) Démonstration de l'origine neurale des cellules à calcitonine du corps ultimobranchial chez l'embryon de poulet. C R Acad Sci (Paris) 270: 2857–2860
LiVolsi VA, Feind CR (1979) Incidental medullary thyroid carcinoma in sporadic hyperparathyroidism. An expansion of the concept of C-cell hyperplasia. Am J Clin Pathol 71: 595–599
Ljungberg O, Nilsson PO (1991) Intermediate thyroid carcinoma in humans and ultimobranchial tumors in bulls: a comparative morphological and immunohistochemical study. Endocr Pathol 2: 24–39
Lloyd RV, Sisson JC, Marangos PJ (1983) Calcitonin, carcinoembryonic antigen and neuron-specific enolase in medullary thyroid carcinoma. An immunohistochemical study. Cancer 51: 2234–2239
Marcus JN, Dise CA, LiVolsi VA (1982) Melanin production in a medullary thyroid carcinoma. Cancer 49: 2518–2526
Martin-Lacave I, Gonzalez-Campora R, Moreno Fernandez A, Sanchez Gallego F, Montero C, Galera-Davidson H (1988) Mucosubstances in medullary carcinoma of the thyroid. Histopathology 13: 55–66
Milhaud G, Moukhtar MS, Bourichon J, Perault AM (1965) Existence et activité de la thyrocalcitonine chez l'homme. C R Acad Sci (Paris) 261: 4513–4516
Min KW, Clemens A, Bell J, Dick H (1988) Malignant peripheral nerve sheath tumor and pheochromcytoma. Arch Pathol Lab Med 112: 266–270
Mizukami Y, Michigishi T, Nonomura A, Nakamura S, Noguchi M, Hashimoto T, Itoh N (1993) Mixed medullary-follicular carcinoma of the thyroid occurring in familial form. Histopathology 22: 284–287
Mulligan LM, Ponder BAJ (1995) Genetic basis of endocrine disease: multiple endocrine neoplasia type 2. J Clin Endocrinol Metab 80:1989–1995
Noel M, Delehaye MC, Segond N, Lasmoles F, Caillou B, Gardet P, Fragu P, Moukhtar MS (1991) Study of calcitonin and thyroglobulin gene expression in human mixed follicular and medullary thyroid carcinoma. Thyroid 1: 249–256
Nonidez JF (1932) The origin of the "parafollicular" cell, a second epithelial component of the thyroid gland. Am J Anat 49: 479–505
Parham DM (1988) Laterally situated neck cysts derived from the embryological remnants of thyroid development. Histopathology 12: 95–98
Pearse AGE (1966) The cytochemistry of the thyroid C cells and their relationship to calcitonin. Proc R Soc Lond [Biol] 164: 478–487
Sambade C, Franssila K, Basilio-de-Oliveira CA, Sobrinho-Simoes M(1990) Mucoepidermoid carcinoma of the thyroid revisited. Surg Pathol 3: 271–280
Schmid KW, Kirchmair R, Ladurner D, Fischer-Colbrie R, Böcker W (1992) Immunohistochemical comparison of chromogranins A and B and secretogranin II with calcitonin and calcito-

nin gene-related peptide expression in normal, hyperplastic and neoplastic C-cells of the human thyroid. Histopathology 21: 225–232
Schröder S, Böcker W, Baisch H, Burk CG, Arps H, Meiners I, Kastendieck H, Heitz PU, Klöppel G (1988) Prognostic factors in medullary thyroid carcinoma. Survival in relation to age, sex, stage, histology, immunocytochemistry, and DNA content. Cancer 61: 806–816
Sobrinho-Simoes M, Sambade C, Nesland JM, Holm R, Damjanov I (1990) Lectin histochemistry and ultrastructure of medullary carcinoma of the thyroid gland. Arch Pathol Lab Med 114: 369–375
Stanton A, Allen-Mersh TG (1984) Is laterally-situated ectopic thyroid tissue always malignant? J R Soc Med 77: 333–334
Tischler AS, Dichter MA, Bailes B, DeLellis RA, Wolfe H (1976) Neural properties of cultured human endocrine cells of proposed neural crest origin. Science 192: 962–964
Williams ED (1966) Histogenesis of medullary carcinoma of the thyroid. J Clin Pathol 19: 114–118
Williams ED (1967) Medullary carcinoma of the thyroid. J Clin Pathol 20: 395–398
Williams ED (1979) The aetiology of thyroid tumours. Clin Endocrinol Metab 8: 193–207
Williams ED, Toyn CE, Harach HR (1989) The ultimobranchial gland and congenital thyroid abnormalities in man. J Pathol 159: 135–141
Wright NA (1990) Endocrine cells in non-endocrine tumours. J Pathol 161: 85–87

Advances in Immunocytochemistry of Thyroid Tumours 1987–1994

B. Jasani

1 Introduction

The history of application of immunocytochemistry to the study of thyroid tumours goes back to the discovery of autoantibodies to thyroglobulin in mid-1950s and the realisation that such autoantibodies as well as heterologous animal antibodies may be used for immunofluorescence tracing of thyroglobulin in normal and neoplastic thyroids. By the early 1970s, the basic idea of using an antibody to trace cell specific antigen was applied to identify parafollicular or C-cell tumours of the thyroid using antibodies to calcitonin (Wolfe et al. 1974). This approach also proved crucial in establishing the existence of familial versus sporadic forms of medullary carcinomas (De Lellis et al. 1979). Since then the use of the more powerful immunoenzyme technology and an increasing variety of cell lineage specific antibodies have proved eminently important in the recognition of mixed

Current Topics in Pathology
Volume 91, K.W. Schmid/W. Böcker (Eds.)

follicular/medullary tumours, anaplastic carcinomas, primary lymphoma, and haemangioendothelioma of thyroid origin. These advances have been reviewed previously by Williams (1986) and Jasani and Newman (1988). The object of this chapter is to give a brief account of the more recently introduced immunocytochemical markers, focusing on their diagnostic and prognostic usefulness in relation to previously established markers of value in differential diagnostic and prognostic analysis of human thyroid tumours. The new and old markers and their respective differential diagnostic and prognostic uses are summarised in Tables 1 and 2. Contributions to improved reliability of thyroid tumour typing, either through the use of better preserved tissue material for analysis, more rigorous sample and case selection criteria, or increased understanding of the underlying molecular and cell biological principles of thyroid tumour growth and behaviour, are also discussed wherever appropriate.

2 Novel Markers in Differential Diagnostic Evaluation of Thyroid Tumours

The advances in differential diagnostic analysis of thyroid tumours have depended critically upon the availability of cell lineage-specific antibody markers. These are listed in Table 1 according to the differential diagnoses they have proved consistently useful in resolving. The newer antibody markers amongst these include those directed at c-erb B2 (a growth factor receptor), calcitonin gene-related peptide (CGRP), laminin, L26 (a pan B-cell antigen), AE1/AE3 (broad-spectrum cytokeratins), HMB 45 (a melanoma-specific antigen), prostate-specific antigen (PSA), KP1 (a pan monocyte/macrophage series cell-specific antigen), and α-smooth muscle actin (α-SMA).

The use of these in combination with previously established set of markers including thyroglobulin (Tg), calcitonin (CT), carcinoembryonic antigen (CEA), leucocyte common antigen (LCA; CD45), and factor VIII-related antigen or von Willebrand factor (F VIII RAG or vWf), have been shown by further studies conducted over the past 7 years to provide adequate panels for resolving the histologically derived differential diagnoses listed in Table 1.

The relative usefulness of these in relation to the individual sets of differential diagnoses resolved is discussed below under separate headings.

2.1 c-erb B2 and Thyroid Follicular vs Papillary Carcinoma

Histopathological criteria for defining thyroid papillary carcinomas should be adequate to distinguish them from follicular carcinomas in all situations except perhaps for the follicular variant of papillary carcinoma, in which the papillary component is either lacking or not so obvious. A number of attempts have been made in the past to produce markers to distinguish the two types of tumours on

Table 1. Immunocytochemical markers useful for differential diagnosis of thyroid tumours

Differential diagnosis	Markers	Key references
1. Follicular vs follicular variant of papillary carcinoma	c-erb B2	HAUGEN et al. (1992)
2. Medullary vs follicular carcinoma		
(a) Follicular vs follicular variant of papillary and/or mixed follicular medullary carcinoma	Tg; CT; metallothionein	HOLM et al. (1989) DE MICCO et al. (1993) SCHMID et al. (1994)
(b) Medullary vs hyalinising trabecular adenoma	Tg; CT; laminin	KATOH et al. (1989)
3. Familial vs sporadic medullary carcinomas	CT; CEA; CGRP	WILLIAMS et al. (1987)
4. Anaplastic carcinoma vs poorly or undifferentiated tumours of the thyroid		
(a) Anaplastic carcinoma vs primary lymphoma of the thyroid	Tg; LCA; L26	SHVERO et al. (1988) WOLF et al. (1992)
(b) Anaplastic carcinoma vs primary and secondary non-lymphomatous tumours of thyroid	Tg; CT; LCA; HMB45; vWf; KP1; α-SMA; AE1/AE3	SHVERO et al. (1988) ORDONEZ et al. (1991)
(c) Metastastic anaplastic carcinoma of the thyroid vs secondaries of unknown primary	Tg; CT; CEA; LCA; PSA	MEYERS and GOODNIGHT (1986) LERTPRASERTSUKE et al. (1990)

histogenetic grounds in the belief that they arise from two distinct subsets of thyroid follicular cells. These efforts have largely been in vain. Current views on the histogenesis of the two types of tumours suggest that they probably arise from a single type of precursor cell but differ histologically and behaviourally because of different sets of oncogenic events leading to their development and progression. Such a hypothesis has been recently put forward by WYNFORD-THOMAS (1993), and it opens up the possibility of using the differential expression of oncogenic products (mainly growth factors and their respective receptors) by these two cancers as a means of distinguishing one from the other on immunocytochemical grounds. The feasibility of this approach is discussed at the end of this chapter.

Amongst a number of growth factor/receptor-specific markers examined by HAUGEN et al. (1992), c-erb B2 was found to be exclusively expressed by papillary carcinomas. This result, though interesting and important, needs to be reproduced in an independent study since this was the first study of its kind. Moreover, the success of the immunostaining was based on the use of frozen sections since the sensitivity in conventional formalin-fixed paraffin sections was lacking. Either the use of a more effective c-erb B2 antibody marker and/or a more sensitive secondary detection system needs to be applied in future studies to obviate this handicap and make the marker useful in the wider context of routine histopathological practice. A recent study conducted to examine this issue on breast carcinoma tissue found commercially available antibody Tab250 (Triton, Thamer Diagnostica Nederlands) to be effective on buffered formalin-fixed paraffin-embedded tissue sections. The antibody gave results comparable to those obtained with the commercial antibody NCLCB11 (Novacostra) on frozen sections as applied by PENAULT-LLORCA et al. (1994).

2.2 CGRP and Familial vs Sporadic Medullary Carcinoma of Thyroid

The distinction between the sporadic and familial forms of medullary carcinomas of the thyroid is based amongst other criteria upon identification of background C-cell hyperplasia in the latter and its absence in the former. Although the nodular form of C-cell hyperplasia is easy to differentiate from normal C cells (occurring mainly in the central portion of the thyroid gland) using immunocytochemistry directed against calcitonin, there are circumstances (e.g. in older patients) where C-cell hyperplasia is nevertheless difficult to discern readily and reliably from the normal type. A number of past studies have therefore attempted to develop markers specific to hyperplastic C cells. These attempts have largely failed. In the late 1980s the discovery of CGRP as a product of an alternatively spliced calcitonin gene in mostly neural tissues and tumours gave new hope in this direction, in the sense that only the neoplastic C cells and their putative precursors the hyperplastic C-cells in a familial setting may aberrently express CGRP. The study, reported by WILLIAMS et al. (1987), was the first to put forward and examine this possibility. However, the authors found normal C cells also to be capable of expressing CGRP, in lower but sufficiently significant amounts to confuse the situation. Since then a number of other studies have confirmed this finding.

2.3 Basement Proteins (Laminin and Type IV Collagen) and Hyalinizing Trabecular Adenoma vs Medullary Carcinoma and Other Thyroid Epithelial Tumours

The amyloid-like substance associated with hyalinising adenoma of the thyroid, together with its trabecular pattern of growth, could pose diagnostic problems with respect to the closely similar features exhibited by medullary carcinoma of the thyroid. KATOH et al. (1989), working on the notion that the amorphous substance may represent overproduction of basement membrane substance, applied laminin as well as collagen type IV-specific antibodies to a small series of diagnostically certain hyalinising trabecular adenomas. They found that this indeed was the case.

Since then they have confirmed the point in a further study (KATOH et al. 1993), in which they examined these antibodies together with an antibody to another basement marker, heparan sulphate. They also included in the study a series of hyperplastic Graves' disease thyroids and follicular and papillary thyroid tumours. They found that whilst laminin and collagen type IV immunostaining gave results of equal specificity and sensitivity, antibody to heparan sulphate produced generally weaker staining. Interestingly, focal deposits of epithelial basement membrane, but much smaller than the lumpy deposits of the hyalinising adenoma, were also observed in follicular adenomas and papillary carcinomas. They concluded that laminin and collagen type IV immunocytochemistry should be used as an aid to the differential diagnosis of primary tumours of thyroid origin showing focal basement membrane accumulations. Furthermore, they noted that, outside the thyroid, overproduction of basement membrane proteins has also been observed in some malignant neoplasms such as adenoid cystic carcinoma and yolk sac tumour. This point has been previously observed by BARSKY et al. (1988).

2.4 L26 (Pan B-Cell Marker) and "Small" Cell Anaplastic Carcinoma vs Lymphoma of the Thyroid

Distinguishing the so-called small cell variant of anaplastic carcinoma from primary lymphoma of the thyroid has been a controversial issue for some time. However, with the advent of the leucocyte common antigen (LCA; CD45) antibody marker, reactive against an epitope stable in formalin-fixed paraffin-embedded tissue substrate, it has been possible to rule out the majority of these types of tumours as being lymphomatous in origin (SHVERO et al. 1988). In a more recent and very rigorously conducted study by WOLF et al. (1992), these findings have been confirmed. In addition, this work has led to the recommendation that L26, an antibody against the formalin-resistant epitope of the cytoplasmic domain of the CD20-defined molecule, should be included as a confirmatory marker to aid the diagnosis. In this context all but two of the 67 histopathologically defined primary thyroid lymphomas were confirmed by WOLF et al. (1992) to be of B-cell origin using this antibody. Furthermore, the antibody proved marginally more sensitive than LCA, which defined only 63/67 tumours as being lymphomatous in origin.

2.5 Pan Cytokeratin, Desmoplakin, HMB 45 (Melanoma Marker), Factor VIII-Related Antigen and KP1 (Pan Macrophage Marker) in the Differential Diagnosis of Anaplastic Carcinomas and Sarcomas of the Thyroid

Spindle or giant cell variants of anaplastic thyroid carcinomas pose several differential diagnostic problems. Thus they may mimic haemangioendotheliomas and other forms of sarcomas, melanomas, or fibrous histiocytic lesions. Recent studies conducted by SHVERO et al. (1988), BELTRAMI et al. (1989) and ORDONEZ et al.

(1991) have shown that the above set of markers is adequate to help resolve this difficulty in most cases.

The pan cytokeratin marker defined by a cocktail of two mouse monoclonal antibodies, AE1/AE3 (SHVERO et al. 1988), and desmoplakin (BELTRAMI et al. 1989), were found to be the two most sensitive markers for identifying epithelial differentiation in spindle or giant cell anaplastic carcinoma variants. Whilst AE1/AE3 worked efficiently on typsinised sections of formalin-fixed paraffin-embedded tissue specimens, desmoplakin appeared to be effective only on frozen sections. The advent of high-temperature antigen retrieval methods and an understanding of their underlying mechanism (BANKFALVI et al. 1994; MORGAN et al. 1994) may prove helpful in developing a technique for revealing this antigen in archival surgical biopsy material.

According to the above studies factor VIII-RAG is effective for confirming the endothelial origin of tumour cells associated with haemangioendotheliomas and the new melanoma-specific marker HMB 45, for unambiguous typing of melanoma metastasis masquerading as an anaplastic carcinoma. Finally, KP1, the pan macrophage marker, should allow identification of many if not all of the giant cells associated with the giant cell anaplastic carcinoma variant as being of reactive histiocytic origin.

2.6 Reappraisal of Thyroglobulin and Calcitonin as Markers in the Differential Diagnosis of Thyroid Tumours

Immunocytochemistry has proved very useful in distinguishing follicular cell tumours from mixed follicular/medullary carcinoma of the thyroid, and in identification of thyroid follicular carcinoma or medullary carcinoma arising as metastases from an unknown primary. A number of recent papers have returned to and reemphasised the important role of immunocytochemistry in resolving these old conundrums of the differential diagnosis of tumours of thyroid origin. The main conclusions of these studies are as summarised below.

2.6.1 Thyroglobulin and Calcitonin in Follicular vs Mixed Follicular/Medullary Carcinoma of Thyroid

The study by DE MICCO et al. (1993) is the most lucid of the recent accounts reviewing histomorphological and immunocytochemical differences between the follicular, mixed follicular/medullary and medullary carcinomas of the thyroid. Through careful choice of diagnostically completely certain cases of medullary thyroid cancer, primary and metastatic tumour tissue from a number of these, and a panel of polyclonal and monoclonal antibodies to thyroglobulin, they obtained convincing evidence to support the notion that the pattern of thyroglobulin and calcitonin expression taken together with the morphological characteristics of the tumour should constitute a sufficient basis for reliable differential diagnosis of these tumour types.

Using diagnostic tissue material available from 19 calcitonin-secreting tumours and 13 secondaries associated with them (2 of them with calcitonin secretory activity), De Micco and colleagues showed that thyroglobulin staining associated with the presence of follicular structures in the middle of the tumour but surrounded by thyroglobulin-negative structures invariably represented entrapped follicles. Similarly, if the tumour cells were positive as an isolated cluster of cells, the staining was likely to be due to an uptake of thyroglobulin degradation products by the the tumour cells from neighbouring entrapped follicles not visible in the sections. Genuine expression of thyroglobulin by tumour cells of medullary carcinoma origin was found in just 2 cases out of the 19. In these cases, the thyroglobulin- as well as calcitonin-positive tumour cells were distributed throughout the tumour, concordant with a mixed trabecular/follicular pattern of histomorphological differentiation, unlike the solid pattern often shown by the pure form of medullary carcinoma. Furthermore, in the lymph node metastases, the thyroglobulin positivity associated with the pure form of medullary carcinoma was shown to be associated with macrophages and not tumour cells.

With these clearly defined guidelines emerging from this study, it should be accepted that the bulk of the thyroglobulin expression in medullary carcinomas (e.g. 35% incidence reported by one study) is focally distributed and due to entrapped follicles or uptake of thyroglobulin by either tumour cells or histiocytic cells. In the light of this postulate, the apparently contradictory observation made by Holm et al. (1989), in their study dealing with 17 cases of sporadic medullary carcinoma with focal areas of thyroglobulin expression, may be explained as follows. They found that extensive analysis under the electron microscope revealed no immunocytochemical evidence of thyroglobulin expression in neurosecretory granule-positive tumour cells. The failure may have been due to general paucity of thyroglobulin-positive cells as revealed under the light microscope, but equally it could have been due to the fact that the isolated clusters of thyroglobulin-positive cells represented entrapped follicles rather than genuine mixed medullary/thyroid follicular tumour cells. This notion is further supported by the fact that all the tumours described by Holm et al. (1989) were histologically of the solid growth pattern and not of the mixed trabecular/follicular pattern which is truly representative of the mixed follicular/C-cell neoplasm.

Recently Schmid et al. (1994) have described fairly consistent expression of immunocytochemically detectable metallothionein using a commercially available monoclonal antibody (E9, Dakopatts Ltd). In striking contrast, this antibody failed to stain normal, hyperplastic or neoplastic C cells. The antibody was therefore found useful in detecting entrapped follicles as well as genuine thyroglobulin-expressing cells in medullary and true mixed medullary/follicular carcinomas. For example, in 4/4 mixed medullary/follicular carcinomas metallothionein staining matched the thyroglobulin-positive areas in semi-adjacent section areas. Also, quite remarkably, individual or clusters of metallothionein-stained cells were very clearly defined and were free of any diffusion artifacts seen for thyroglobulin. Tumour areas positive for calcitonin and/or CGRP were universally negative for metallothionein. Metallothionein may therefore be used as a helpful marker to thyroglobulin in diagnosis of mixed medullary/follicular carcinomas.

2.6.2 Thyroglobulin in Differential Diagnosis of Metastasis of Unknown Primary

The study by Meyers and Goodnight (1986) provides proof that immunocytochemistry of thyroglobulin in a tissue biopsy taken from a metastatic tumour is more reliable than radionuclide scanning for diagnostic identification of a new or previously resected thyroid primary. Their work and that of Lertprasertsuke et al. (1990) support the viewpoint that immunocytochemical screening is by far the cheaper and safer of the two alternatives, and re-emphasise the old adage that identification in the case of a patient with a tumour of unknown primary, of treatable varieties of tumours including lymphomas, germ cell tumours, and adenocarcinomas of thyroid, ovaries, breast or prostate, is a highly desirable adjunct to proper management of such patients.

3 Markers in Prognostic Evaluation of Thyroid Tumours

Prognostic analysis is aimed at identification of histological and molecular traits of a tumour relating to its potential clinical behaviour, in particular its capacity to grow relentlessly and rapidly, to recur and to invade locally or extensively. All these features of tumour behaviour are associated with a significant shortening of the patient's survival span. It is therefore important from the point of view of proper patient management that these features of a tumour are recognised and appropriately aggressive treatment instituted.

What follows is a brief review of the evolving use of immunocytochemistry in the prognostic analysis of thyroid epithelial tumours. The principal antibody markers attempted so far and their most significant contributions are summarised in Table 2. As for medullary thyroid carcinomas, although a wide variety of markers have been applied for prognostic classification, none of these have proved sufficently effective for the purpose, as indicated by the studies of Franc et al. (1987), Takami et al. (1988), Schröder et al. (1988) and Scopsi et al. (1990). Hence, these are not included for further consideration below. Also, the review as a whole is restricted to antibody markers which are applicable to formalin-fixed, paraffin-embedded tissues sections prepared routinely in a clinical setting.

3.1 Markers of Value in Differentiation of Follicular Adenomas from Follicular Carcinomas

An adenoma may be considered by definition to be inherently incapable of metastasis or recurrence, whereas a carcinoma possesses both these attributes. Distinction of a thyroid follicular adenoma from a well-differentiated carcinoma is therefore important but can be difficult as it depends solely upon finding evidence of capsular or vascular invasion. For this purpose multiple blocks through the capsular region of the tumour are necessary – a condition which may not be always satisfied readily. An alternative method is therefore highly desirable. So far no

Table 2. Applications of immunocytochemistry in prognostic analysis of thyroid epithelial tumours

Application	Antibody marker	Principal references
Differentiation of thyroid follicular adenoma vs carcinoma	Monoclonal anti-ras p21 (MoAb RAP-50)	Mizukami et al. (1988)
	Monoclonal anti-thyroid peroxidase, TPO (MoAb 47)	De Micco et al. (1991)
Assessment of malignant potential of differentiated thyroid follicular and papillary carcinomas	Polyclonal anti-human TGF-β	Jasani et al. (1990)
	Polyclonal anti-thyroglobulin, T4 & T3 antibodies	Batge et al. (1992)
	Monoclonal anti-oestrogen receptor (MoAb H222)	Hiasa et al. (1993)
	Monoclonal anti-epithelial membrane antigen (MoAb M613)	Yamamoto et al. (1992)
	Monoclonal anti-proliferating cell nuclear antigen (MoAb PC10)	Mizukami et al. (1993)
	Monoclonal anti-epidermal growth factor	Mizukami et al. (1993)
	Polyclonal anti-p53 (CM10)	Wright et al. (1993)
	Monoclonal anti-metallothionein (E9)	Schmid et al. (1994)

particular immunocytochemical marker has proved entirely satisfactory in distinguishing the two types of tumour entity. Nevertheless, studies by Mizukami et al. (1988) and De Micco et al. (1991) give interesting accounts of immunocytochemically definable oncogene expression and antigenic differences between follicular adenomas and carcinomas.

The work done by Mizukami et al. (1988) related to immunocytochemical study of ras p21 oncogene product expression in a large series of normal, hyperplastic, benign and malignant thyroid follicular epithelial tissues. They used a mouse monoclonal RAP-5 generated against a synthetic peptide corresponding to amino acid position 10–17 of the ras p21 protein. With this antibody they found cytoplasmic expression of the ras p21 protein in all grades of thyroid lesions, but the apical cell surface staining was found to be almost exclusively restricted to 4/4 follicular carcinomas and 33/34 papillary carcinomas studied. Thus, only 1/13 simple follicular adenomas and 1/24 goitrous or hyperplastic thyroid lesions produced some staining, and this was at the most weak in intensity. The authors commented that at the practical level immunocytochemically detectable apical surface staining of ras p21 protein may be used for differentiation of a follicular adenoma from a follicular carcinoma.

A mutation of H-, K-, and N-*ras* gene has been found to be a frequent initiating event (i.e. in about 60% of cases) in thyroid follicular cell oncogenesis. Whether the apical surface expression of p21 ras protein is associated with a particular subset of *ras* gene mutations needs to be investigated.

The work by DE MICCO et al. (1991) related to mouse monoclonal antibodies to purified thyroid peroxidase, TPO (formerly referred to as the thyroid microsomal antigen). They found antibody MoAb 47 to give consistently strong staining of the adenomas and only weak to negative results for the majority of papillary (39/43) and follicular carcinomas (15/22). They also noticed a focal lack of TPO expression in some adenomas and focal expression of it in some follicular carcinomas. They concluded that this type of staining may be representative of progression towards preinvasive and more malignant stages of thyroid follicular carcinogenesis. Hence, the antibody may be useful for sub-categorisation of adenomas as well as well-differentiated thyroid follicular carcinomas into their more malignant variants.

The antibody may also have application in cytologic identification of poorly differentiated follicular carcinoma, which would be expected to be uniformly negative for the antibody staining. However, as pointed out by DE MICCO et al. (1991), the TPO staining in normal thyroid tissue surrounding a proportion of large, poorly differentiated follicular carcinomas was found to be negative. This potentially confusing finding, according to these authors, may be due to a release of soluble factors capable of modifying TPO expression in normal tissue and/or impeding the MoAb 47 binding.

3.2 Immunocytochemical Markers in Assessment of Malignant Potential of Thyroid Follicular and Papillary Carcinomas

Follicular, papillary and anaplastic carcinomas of the thyroid constitute the three major types of malignant tumours arising from the thyroid follicular epithelium. Whilst a diagnosis of an anaplastic variant of thyroid carcinoma automatically connotes a poor prognosis, the follicular and papillary carcinomas do not seem to be very homogenous in their prognostic outcomes even when lymph node or distant metastases are taken into consideration. This has necessitated a search for more discriminatory markers of prognosis in these types of tumours. Recent advances in immunocytochemical technology, and our increasing understanding of the cell and molecular biological basis of thyroid epithelial cancer, have led a number of workers in the field to examine the value of immunocytochemical markers based on these novel techniques and concepts. The most salient findings to date of this new approach are summarised below.

The possible role of changes in immunocytochemically detectable TGF-β expression in the multistage development of thyroid follicular cell cancer has been examined by JASANI et al. (1990). In this study an antibody directed against the amino-terminal 30 amino acids of human TGF-β_1 was applied to a series of benign thyroid lesions and follicular, papillary and anaplastic thyroid carcinomas. None of the seven thyroid follicular adenomas nor normal thyroid epithelium studied showed any positive staining. In the cancer group no significant correlation was found between TGF-β immunostaining and pathological grade or clinical stage. However, a significant correlation was noted between TGF-β expression and a specific mutation of the H-*ras* gene oncogene (codon 61, Gln→Arg) in the follicular carcinoma subcategory. The overall data suggested that a major alteration in TGF-β expression is associated specifically with the malignant stage of thyroid follicular cell carcinogenesis.

It may be expected that as thyroid follicular tumours become more and more malignant, the lack of histological differentiation may be accompanied or even preceded by a loss of antigens associated with thyroid function, e.g. thyroglobulin, T4 and T3. Remarkably, in a study by Batge et al. (1992), 97% (i.e. 60/62 cases) of recurrent or metastastic thyroid follicular tumours were found to express thyroglobulin and T4 even though positive radio-iodine was limited to just 44%. Interestingly, only 6% (4/62) of the tumours expressed T3, presumably due to type I 5'-deiodinase activity associated with malignant neoplastic transformation. In summary, the study has helped to show that the immunocytochemically detectable thyroglobulin and T4 expression is independent of malignant potential or structural pattern of growth in differentiated thyroid follicular carcinomas.

The incidence of thyroid epithelial tumours is nearly three-fold greater in females than in males, and sex hormones are known to exert a strong influence on the growth-promoting effects of thyroid-stimulating hormone (TSH). This led Hiasa et al. (1993) to examine oestrogen receptor (ER) status in normal, goitrous and neoplastic human thyroid tissue. They successfully applied the established marker of ER in frozen tissue sections, the H222 mouse monoclonal antibody belonging to the ER-ICA kit (Abbott Laboratories), to formalin-fixed paraffin sections pretreated with 10% protease applied for 10 min at 37°C. Applying this modified approach to over 300 thyroid specimens, they found a consistent loss of ER positivity associated with lesions showing increasing proliferative potential. Thus, nodular goitre gave the highest incidence of positivity at 58.9%, compared to the 33.8%, 30.4%, 16.5% and 0% rates observed for thyroid adenoma and follicular, papillary and anaplastic carcinomas, respectively. The overall data taken together with similar findings of other workers in the field suggest that down-regulation or loss of ER is associated with increased malignant potential of neoplastic thyroid epithelial lesions.

Papillary carcinoma is the most common type of thyroid malignancy and is characterised by a slow growth pattern and long-term survival. The tumour is nevertheless associated with mortality in a small but significant proportion of cases. For example, 6.5% of 859 cases studied by McConahey et al. (1986) at the Mayo Clinic were found to die of the disease. Although the age and gender of the patient, microscopic type, tumour size and initial extent of tumour spread may all contribute to the overall bad prognosis, cell biological parameters outside the scope of clinicopathological assessment may also be important. To this effect Yamamoto et al. (1992) have applied on an empirical basis antibodies to epithelial membrane antigen (EMA), cytokeratin and vimentin to a series of papillary thyroid carcinomas with and without evidence of distance metastases. They found an increase in EMA positivity of the tumour cells to be significantly associated with a tendency of a tumour to metastasise. They suggested that this may be related to the

EMA's recognised capacity to prevent cell-cell contact inhibition, and accordingly the EMA-positive tumour cells may spread in a less constrained way. No similar or any other type of association of cytokeratin or vimentin overexpression was found with the clinicopathologically definable malignant potential of the tumour.

MIZUKAMI et al. (1993), on the other hand, studied on a more rational basis epidermal growth factor (EGF, a 53 amino acid residue polypeptide) with a known capacity to stimulate proliferation and differentiation of a variety of epithelial cells. They also examined proliferating cell nuclear antigen (PCNA) as an acknowledged marker of the proliferation potential of a tumour cell population. Both these markers were applied in relation to histologically defined prognostic subtypes (i.e. well-differentiated, follicular and trabecular variants, respectively) of papillary thyroid carcinomas derived from 50 cases.

Their use of PCNA marker in addition to the conventional mitotic counts was also motivated by the the difficulty of differentiating mitotic figures from pyknotic nuclei. The recent introduction of the commercially available monoclonal antibody PC10, capable of detecting PCNA in formalin-fixed, paraffin-embedded tissue sections, was helpful in this study. However, despite these favourable points no significant association was found between mitotic counts, PCNA expression and DNA ploidy status and histologic subtypes of papillary thyroid carcinomas. This finding is also in keeping with the data of SHIMIZU et al. (1993), who compared PCNA expression in 17 well-differentiated versus 7 poorly differentiated papillary thyroid carcinomas. SHIMIZU et al. nevertheless emphasised that a significantly greater level of PCNA expression is consistently associated with the nuclei of follicular adenoma and adenomatous goitre compared to normal thyroid epithelium, on the one hand, and papillary thyroid carcinomas compared to normal thyroid, adenomatous goitre and follicular adenoma tissue, on the other.

MIZUKAMI et al. (1993) found a significant relationship between overexpression of EGF and histologic features associated with poor prognosis, in particular the trabecular growth pattern of papillary thyroid carcinoma. Their previous study had already noted in addition a direct correlation between EGF overexpression and recurrences of papillary thyroid carcinoma (MIZUKAMI et al. 1991). The overall data, which are also supported by findings of GORGOULIS et al. (1992), suggest that combined overexpression of EGF and its receptor is likely to be associated with a more aggressive course of the disease.

Another marker that may be used for identifying tumours with a more aggressive growth tendency is p53, a product of tumour suppressor gene, *TP53*. Thus, point mutations in the *TP53* gene have been found to be restricted to poorly differentiated and anaplastic thyroid carcinomas (DONGHI et al. 1993; WYNFORD-THOMAS 1993). It is also possible to use immunocytochemistry directed at p53 protein as an in situ method for detecting *TP53* gene mutations. This is because mutations in the *TP53* gene often result in overexpression of p53 due to the resistance of the mutated protein against degradation. WRIGHT et al. (1993) has used this approach successfully on formalin-fixed, paraffin-embedded tissue sections, thereby opening up the possibility of applying this approach in a routine clinical setting in the future.

Recently, SCHMID et al. (1993) and ZELGER et al. (1993) have shown immunocytochemically detectable metallothionein overexpression in human breast carcinomas and melanomas to be a consistent marker of poor prognosis in these tumours. The application of this marker to the study of a wide variety of thyroid neoplastic and non-neoplastic lesions has also shown a similar association (SCHMID et al. 1994). Thus papillary carcinomas were found to show pronounced expression only in the less differentiated variants. However, further work needs to be done to elucidate a possible relationship between metallothionein overexpression and clinical course in malignant thyroid follicular tumours.

3.3 Prospects for More Rational Prognostic Markers Based Upon Recent Improved Understanding of the Molecular Genetics of Thyroid Cancer

Over the past 7 years a dramatic improvement in our understanding of the molecular events accompanying and/or leading to thyroid follicular cell tumour progression has been made. The most salient of these have been highlighted in a recent review by WYNFORD-THOMAS (1993). It appears that the development and progression of thyroid follicular tumours is associated with a more or less sequential series of mutations in a small subset of growth-stimulatory oncogenes and growth-inhibitory tumour suppressor genes, making it feasible to use precisely defined associations of genotypic and phenotypic abnormalities as a rational basis for prognostic analysis of thyroid follicular tumours.

The five genes accounting for the carcinogenesis of nearly 60% of human thyroid follicular tumours include *gsp*, *ras*, *trk*, *ret* and *TP53*. Mutations causing activation of the gsp and ras genes on one hand and the *trk* and *ret* genes on the other are associated with increased growth potential of the follicular adenomas and carcinomas and of the papillary carcinomas, respectively, whilst those involving the *TP53* are linked to conversion of a low-grade to more aggressive high-grade thyroid follicular carcinoma.

Since the mutations in the *ras*, *ret* and *TP53* genes are frequently associated with increased expression of their respective protein products, the available antibodies to these proteins should allow immunocytochemical detection of the protein overexpression in the context of routinely prepared tumour tissue. However, immunocytochemical positivity of these proteins per se has not been found to constitute sufficient evidence of gene mutation in individual cases, as mechanisms other than gene mutation may also lead to their overexpression. The antibodies have also been found not to be able to distinguish mutated gene product from the native protein. These difficulties have so far therefore prevented realisation of the full potential of this approach in relation to prognostic analysis of thyroid tumours. Further work is needed to resolve such difficulties.

Acknowledgements. The help of Mr. Steve Pritchard, Deputy Librarian, University of Wales College of Medicine, Cardiff, and Mark Edwards, Sixth Form Pupil, Radyr Comprehensive School, Cardiff, is gratefully acknowledged in relation to information retrieval needed for this review.

References

Bankfalvi A, Navabi H, Bier B, Böcker W, Jasani B, Schmid KW (1994) Wet autoclave pretreatment for antigen retrieval in diagnostic immunocytochemistry. J Pathol 174: 223–228

Barsky SH, Layfield L, Varki N, Bhuta S (1988) Two human tumours with high basement membrane-producing potential. Cancer 61: 1798–1806

Batge B, Dralle H, Padberg B, von Herbay B, Schröder S (1992) Histology and immunocytochemistry of differentiated thyroid carcinomas do not predict radio-iodine uptake: a clinicopathological study of 62 recurrent or metastatic tumours. Virchows Archiv [A] 421: 521–526

Beltrami CA, Criante P, Di Loreto C (1989) Immunocytochemistry of anaplastic carcinoma of thyroid gland. Appl Pathol 7: 122–133

De Lellis RA, Nunnemacher G, Bitman WR et al (1979) C-cell hyperplasia and medullary thyroid carcinoma in the rat. An immunohistochemical and ultrastructural analysis. Lab Invest 40: 140–153

De Micco C, Ruf J, Chrestian M-A, Gros N, Henry J-F, Carayon P (1991) Immunohistochemical study of thyroid peroxidase in normal, hyperplastic, and neoplastic human thyroid tissues. Cancer 67: 3036–3041

De Micco C, Chapel F, Dor A-M, Garcia S, Ruf J, Carayon P, Henry J-F, Lebreuil G (1993) Thyroglobulin in medullary thyroid carcinoma: immunohistochemical study with polyclonal and monoclonal antibodies. Hum Pathol 24: 256–262

Donghi R, Longoni A, Piloti S, Michieli P, Porta GD, Pierotti MA (1993) Gene p53 mutations are restricted to poorly differentiated and undifferentiated carcinomas of the thyroid gland. J Clin Invest 91: 1753–1760

Franc B, Caillou B, Carrier AM, Dutrieux N, Floquet J, Houcke M, Justrabo E, Lange F, Rigaud C, Schwartz A, Viennet M, Lebodic MF (1987) Immunohistochemistry in medullary thyroid carcinoma: prognosis and distinction between hereditary and sporadic tumours. Henry Ford Hosp Med J 35: 139–142

Gorgoulis V, Aninos D, Priftis CH, Evagelopoulou C, Karameris A, Kanavaros P, Spandidos DA (1992) Expression of epidermal growth factor, transforming growth factor-alpha and epidermal growth factor receptor in thyroid tumours. In Vivo 6: 291–296

Haugen DRF, Akslen LA, Varhaug, Lillehaug JR (1992) Expression of c-erb-2 protein in papillary thyroid carcinomas. Br J Cancer 65: 832–837

Hiasa Y, Nishioka H, Kitahori Y, Yane K, Nakaoka S, Ohshima M, Konishi K, Kitamura M, Matsunaga T (1993) Immunohistochemical analysis of estrogen receptors in 313 paraffin section cases of human thyroid tissue. Oncology 50: 132–136

Holm R, Farrants GW, Nesland JM, Sobrinho-Simoes M, Jorgensen OG, Johannessen JV (1989) Ultrastuctural and electron immunohistochemical features of medullary thyroid carcinoma. Virchows Arch [A] 414: 375–384

Jasani B, Newman GR (1988) Application of immunocytochemistry to thyroid tumours. In: Wynford-Thomas D, Williams ED (eds) Thyroid tumours. Molecular basis of pathogenesis. Churchill Livingstone, Edinburgh, pp 140–147

Jasani B, Wyllie FS, Wright PA, Lemoine NR, Williams ED, Wynford-Thomas D (1990) Immunocytochemically detectable TGF-beta associated with malignancy in thyroid epithelial neoplasia. Growth Factors 2: 149–155

Katoh R, Jasani B, Williams ED (1989) Hyalinizing trabecular adenoma of the thyroid. A report of three cases with immunohistochemical and ultrastructural studies. Histopathology 15: 211–224

Katoh R, Muramatsu A, Kawaoi A, Komiyama A, Suzuki K, Hemmi A, Katayama S (1993) Alteration of the basement membrane in human thyroid diseases: an immunohistochemical study of type IV collagen, laminin and heparan sulphate proteoglycan. Virchows Arch [A] 423: 417–424

Lertprasertsuke N, Kakuda K, Satoh S, Tada N, Samura Y (1990) Rectal carcinoid tumour metastasing to the thyroid and pancreas: an autopsy case exploiting immunohistochemistry for differentiation from tumours involving multiple endocrine organs. Acta Pathol Jpn 40: 352–360

Mason DY, Comans-Bitter M, Cordell JL et al (1990) Antibody L26 recognises an intracellular epitope on the B-cell associated CD20 antigen. Am J Pathol 136: 1215–1222

McConahey WM, Hay ID, Woolner LB, van Heerden JA, Taylor WF (1986) Papillary thyroid cancer treated at Mayo Clinic, 1946 through 1970: initial manifestations, pathologic findings, therapy, and outcome. Mayo Clin Proc 61: 978–996

Meyers FJ, Goodnight J (1986) Identification of unsuspected thyroid carcinoma using immunoperoxidase for thyroglobulin. Am J Med 81: 177–179

Mizukami Y, Nonomura A, Hashimoto T, Terahata S, Matsubara F, Michigishi T, Noguchi M (1988) Immunohistochemical demonstration of ras p21 oncogene product in normal, benign, and malignant human thyroid tissues. Cancer 61: 873–880

Mizukami Y, Nonomura A, Hashimoto T et al (1991) Immunohistochemical demonstration of epidermal growth factor and c-myc oncogene product in normal, benign and malignant thyroid tissues. Histopathology 18: 11–18

Mizukami Y, Nonomura A, Michigishi T, Noguchi M, Nakamura S, Hashimoto T (1993) Tumour proliferation markers in papillary thyroid carcinomas: correlation with histologic subtypes. Anticancer Res 13: 267–272

Morgan JM, Navabi H, Schmid KW, Jasani B (1994) Possible role of tissue-bound calcium ions in citrate-mediated high temperature antigen retrieval. J Pathol 174: 301–307

Ordonez NG, El-Naggar AK, Hickey RC, Samaan NA (1991) Anaplastic thyroid carcinoma. Immunocytochemical study of 32 cases. Am J Clin Pathol 96: 15–24

Penault-Llorca F, Adelaide J, Houvenaeghel G, Hassoun J, Birnbaum D, Jaquemier J (1994) Optimization of immunohistochemical detection of ERBB2 in human breast cancer. J Pathol 173: 65

Schmid KW, Ellis IO, Gee JMW, Darke BM, Lees WE, Kay J, Cryer A, Stark JM, Hittmair A, Öfner D, Dunser M, Margreiter R, Daxenbichler G, Nicholson RI, Bier B, Böcker W, Jasani B (1993) Presence and possible significance of immunocytochemically demonstrable metallothionein overexpression in primary ductal carcinoma of the breast. Virchows Arch [A] 322: 153–159

Schmid KW, Greeff M, Hittmair A, Tötsch M, Öfner D, Dockhorn-Dwornizak B, Böcker W, Jasani B (1994) Metallothionein expression in normal, hyperplastic, and neoplastic thyroid follicular and parafollicular C-cells using monoclonal anti-metallothionein antibody E9. Endocr Pathol 5: 114–122

Schröder S, Böcker W, Baisch H, Burk CG, Arps H, Meiners I, Kastendieck H, Heitz PU, Klöppel G (1988) Prognostic factors in medullary thyroid carcinomas. Survival in relation to age, sex, stage, histology, immunocytochemistry, and DNA content. Cancer 61: 806–816

Scopsi L, Pilotti S, Rike F (1990) Immunocytochemical localization and identification of members of the pancreatic polypeptide (PP)-fold family in human thyroid C cells and medullary carcinomas. Regul Pept 30: 89–104

Shimizu T, Usuda N, Yamada T, Sugenoya A, Iida F (1993) Proliferative activity of human thyroid tumors evaluated by proliferating cell nuclear antigen/cyclin immunohistochemical studies. Cancer 71: 2807–2812

Shvero J, Gal R, Avidor I, Hadar T, Kessler E (1988) Anaplastic thyroid canrcinoma. A clinical, histologic, and immunohistochemical study. Cancer 62: 319–325

Takami H, Bessho T, Kameya T, Mimura T, Ito K, Abe O, Hosoda Y, Shikata J-I (1988) Immunohistochemical study of medullary thyroid carcinoma: relationship of clinical features to prognostic factors in 36 patients. World J Surg 12: 572–579

Tötsch M, Dobler G, Feichtinger H, Sandbichler P, Ladurner D, Schmid KW (1990) Malignant hemagioendothelioma of the thyroid. Its immunohistochemical discrimination from undifferentiated thyroid carcinoma. Am J Surg Pathol 14: 69–74

Williams ED (1986) Immunocytochemistry in the diagnosis of thyroid diseases. In: Polak JM, Van Noorden S (eds) Immunocytochemistry: modern methods and applications, 2nd edn. Wright, Bristol, pp 533–546

Williams ED, Ponder BJ, Craig RK (1987) CGRP in C-cells and medullary carcinoma. Clin Endocrinol (Oxf) 27: 104–107

Wolf BC, Sheahan K, DeCoste D, Variakojis D, Alpern HD, Haselow RE (1992) Immunohistochemical analysis of small cell tumors of the thyroid gland: an Easter Cooperative Oncology Group Study. Hum Pathol 23: 1252–1261

Wolfe HJ, Voelkil EF, Tashjian AH Jr (1974) Distribution of calcitonin containing cells in normal human thyroid gland: a correlation of morphology with peptide content. J Clin Endocrinol Metab 38: 688–694

Wright PA, Jasani B, Newman GR, Schmid KW, Wynford-Thomas D (1993) p53 immunopositivity is a late event in human thyroid tumorigenesis (Abstr). J Pathol 169: 176

Wynford-Thomas D (1993) Molecular genetics of thyroid cancer. TEM 4: 224–231

Yamamoto Y, Izumi K, Otsuka H (1992) An immunohistochemical study of epithelial membrane antigen, cytokeratin, and vimentin in papillary thyroid carcinoma. Recognition of lethal and favourable prognostic types. Cancer 70: 2326–2333

Zelger B, Hittmair A, Schir M, Öfner C, Öfner D, Fritsch PO, Böcker W, Jasani B, Schmid KW (1993) Immunohistochemically demonstrated metallothionein expression in malignant melanoma. Histopathology 23: 257–264

Minimally Invasive Follicular Thyroid Carcinoma: A Clinico-pathological Study

K.W. Schmid, M. Tötsch, D. Öfner, W. Böcker, and D. Ladurner

1 Introduction

According to the updated WHO classification of thyroid tumours (Hedinger et al. 1988), follicular thyroid carcinomas are divided into two prognostically relevant subgroups, minimally invasive and widely invasive follicular carcinoma. Unlike widely invasive follicular carcinoma, which can be clinically and surgically recognized as a cancer, minimally invasive follicular carcinoma can be diagnosed only by the pathologist.

Macroscopically, minimally invasive follicular carcinoma resembles a follicular adenoma. The lesions are encapsulated and well defined. The only slight hint of malignancy may be the thickness of the tumour capsule. Follicular carcinoma tends sometimes to be surrounded by a thick-walled capsule (Evans 1984).

Microscopically, minimally invasive follicular carcinoma again resembles benign follicular adenoma. The lesions may show a normo- and/or microfollicular and/or a trabecular pattern. In most cases the follicles are regular, small and round. There are no reliable cellular features to distinguish minimally invasive follicular carcinomas from follicular adenomas. Whatever the histological and cytological architecture in the centre of the lesions looks like, however, the area of interest for the pathologist lies in the tumour capsule thyroid interface.

The criteria for the diagnosis of a minimally invasive follicular carcinoma are invasion of the capsule, invasion through the capsule, and invasion into veins in or beyond the tumour capsule. However, in order to substantiate one or more than one of these criteria at least ten tissue blocks of the tumour capsule thyroid interface should be investigated (Kahn and Perzin 1983; Lang et al. 1986; LiVolsi 1990).

Since a lot of effort is put in by the pathologist to the diagnosis or exclusion of minimally invasive follicular carcinoma, it seems to be of special interest to inves-

Current Topics in Pathology
Volume 91, K.W. Schmid/W. Böcker (Eds.)

tigate the clinical outcome of patients with minimally invasive follicular carcinoma. Is one of the diagnostic criteria statistically more often associated with the development of metastases and/or tumour recurrence? We re-examined the cases of minimally invasive follicular carcinomas diagnosed between 1970 and 1987 at the Department of Pathology, University of Innsbruck, Austria, in order to determine whether one of the histological criteria of minimally invasive follicular carcinoma may be more often found in cases with the development of tumour recurrence and/or metastases.

2 Materials and Methods

Between 1970 and 1987, 324 follicular carcinomas of the thyroid were diagnosed at the Department of Pathology, University of Innsbruck, Austria. Two hundred and five (63.3%) of these tumours were widely invasive, 119 (36.7%) minimally invasive. The follow-up data of all 119 patients with minimally invasive tumours were available for this study; the mean observation period was 9.2 years (8 months to 24 years).

3 Results

3.1 Clinical Presentation and Surgical Treatment

The male:female ratio of patients with minimally invasive carcinomas was 1:4.7. The mean age of patients was 44.8 years (range 23–87 years). Seventy-eight (65.5%) tumours were pT2, 41 (34.5%) pT3 tumours. Two patients with pT3 tumours had distant matastases at diagnosis. None of the tumours in this series was smaller than 1 cm in diameter (pT1) or extended beyond the thyroid capsule (pT4). After histological diagnosis, surgical treatment comprised complete thyroidectomy or lobectomy and subtotal lobectomy of the contralateral lobe in 94 cases (79%); in 25 cases (21%) only thyroid resection was performed. All patients with an uneventful clinical course so far have been followed up for at least 7 years.

3.2 Histological Features

The histological diagnosis of a minimally invasive carcinoma was made in 28/119 cases (23.5%) on the basis of invasion beyond the tumour capsule, in 53 cases (44.5%) on the basis of invasion into one or more than one vein located in or beyond the tumour capsule, and in 38 cases (32%) on the basis of both vascular and capsular invasion.

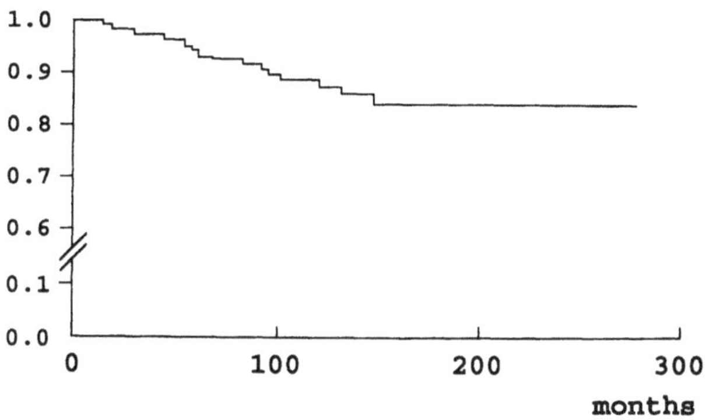

Fig. 1. Kaplan-Meier curve of patients with minimally invasive follicular carcinoma of the thyroid, showing the tumour-free survival of the 119 patients of the preset series

3.3 Follow-Up Data

Sixteen patients (13.4%) developed matastases and/or local tumour recurrence (Fig. 1); 7 (5.9%) died during follow-up. The male : female ratio of these 16 patients was 1 : 3, the mean age 60.2 years (range 40–87 years). Nine of 94 patients (9.6%; mean age 52.1 years) developed matastases or local tumour recurrence after thyroidectomy, 7/25 (28%; mean age 66.3 years) after thyroid resection [$\chi^2 = 4.3$ (contin. corr.); $p < 0.05$].

Tumour recurrence and/or development of matastases occurred in 2/28 (7.1%) patients with invasion exclusively through the tumour capsule, in 8/53 patients (15%) with only vascular invasion, and in 6/38 cases (15.7%) in which both diagnostic criteria could be demonstrated. Thus tumour recurrence and/or metastasis occurred in 14/91 patients (15.4%) with vascular invasion, and in 9/66 patients (13.6%) with capsular invasion. Of the two patients who had distant metastases at diagnosis, one showed vascular and one vascular and capsular invasion.

Tumour recurrence and/or metastasis occurred in the two patients with exclusively capsular invasion after 83 and 68 months, respectively; the second of these patients is still alive (124 months follow-up). In patients with only vascular invasion, tumour recurrence or metastases were detected after a mean period of 47.2 months (range 5–102 months); in patients with vascular and capsular invasion the mean period was 49.8 months (range 8–98 months).

4 Discussion

In (iodine-deficient) endemic goitre areas, follicular thyroid carcinoma constitutes up to 40% of thyroid cancers (Hofstädter 1980; Williams 1980; Schmid et al.

1989; KOBER et al. 1990), whereas it occurs less frequently (5%–20%) in non-endemic-goitre areas (MENDELSOHN 1988; SCHRÖDER 1988; LIVOLSI 1990; MURRAY 1991). The minimally invasive (encapsulated) type accounts for up to 42% of follicular carcinomas (SCHRÖDER et al. 1984; SCHRÖDER 1988). The biological behaviour differs significantly from that of widely invasive follicular carcinoma; the 10-year survival rates are 70%–100% for the minimally invasive type and 25%–50% for the widely invasive type (DONIACH 1978; HOFSTÄDTER 1980; HOFSTÄDTER and UNTERKIRCHER 1980; LADURNER and HOFSTÄDTER 1983; FRANSSILA et al. 1985; SCHRÖDER et al. 1984; SCHRÖDER 1988).

The essentially normal survival of patients with a diagnosis of minimally invasive follicular carcinoma based on borderline histological invasion indicates the need for unequivocal evidence of invasion to establish the diagnosis of carcinoma (HEDINGER et al. 1988). The diagnosis of encapsulated follicular carcinoma thus depends, after careful histologic assessment, on its hallmarks, i.e. vascular invasion *into* veins and/or invasion *through* the capsule (LIVOLSI 1990). The recognition of capsular and vascular invasion in minimally invasive carcinoma, however, is frequently more difficult in practice than it is in theory. The criteria for the identification of vascular and capsular invasion are debated and poorly defined (KAHN and PERZIN 1983; FRANSSILA et al. 1985).

In our experience the diagnosis of minimally invasive follicular carcinoma should only be made if the following criteria are met:

1. For vascular invasion:
   - A tumour plug or ployp in a subendothelial location within a vessel in or beyond the tumour capsule
   - Tumour thrombus usually but not necessarily covered by endothelium
   - Tumour thrombus not attached to the vessel wall, so the point of invasion into the vein has not to be detected
2. For capsular invasion:
   - Penetration of the tumour through the capsule deflecting the collagen fibers of the capsule
   - Contact of the tumour with the surrounding normal thyroid parenchyma
   - Concomitant vascular invasion not required even if matastases are already present at the time of diagosis

Tumour plugs found within the capillaries of the tumour itself are apparently not associated with malignant behaviour (FRANSSILA et al. 1985) and thus have no prognostic or diagnostic relevance.

In the present series vascular invasion and combined vascular and capsular invasion was twice as frequently (15%) associated with the development of tumour recurrence and/or metastasis than invasion through the tumour capsule alone; these findings are in accordance with those of an earlier study (SCHRÖDER et al. 1984). In previous reports, of patients with only capsular invasion, 1/7 (KAHN and PERZIN 1983) and 3/7 respectively (EVANS 1984) had metastases, and in the latter series metastases were already present in all three cases at initial diagnosis.

How many tissue blocks are needed to adequately prove or rule out invasion in an encapsulated follicular tumour? For practical reasons most authors recommend ten tissue blocks as representative of the tumour capsule thyroid interface

(Franssila et al. 1985; Lang et al. 1986; LiVolsi 1990). Since malignancy is more easily demonstrated in larger lesions, ten blocks will cover at least 50% of the tumour mass in pT2 tumours. Like others (LiVolsi 1990), we believe that significant cancer will probably not be missed if ten blocks are carefully examined.

Due to the small number of patients with tumour recurrence and/or metastases in the present series, we cannot comment upon a possible significant influence of vascular or capsular invasion on the period before recurrence or development of metastases. No published data are available on 20- to 30-year follow-up of large numbers of patients with the diagnosis of minimally invasive follicular carcinoma. The majority of recurrences or metastases will appear within 5 years after operation; however, metastases have been described in patients with the diagnosis of an encapsulated follicular carcinoma as much as 24 years before the secondary lesion occurred (LiVolsi 1990). Our results show that adequate surgical treatment is required even in cases of minimally invasive follicular carcinomas. Local tumour recurrence and/or metastatic development was statistically significantly more often associated with thyroid resection than with complete or subtotal thyroidectomy ($p < 0.05$).

The term "atypical adenoma" is currently used to describe a highly cellular tumour with unusual histologic appearance. The irregular architectural and/or cytological patterns of these tumours strongly suggest the possibility of malignancy but after extensive histological examination lack evidence of invasion. Follow-up studies of patients with "atypical adenomas" have shown that these tumours behave in a benign fashion without development of metastases or recurrences (Hazard and Kenyon 1954; Lang et al. 1980, 1986; F. Hofstädter, personal communication). However, as already stated for minimally invasive follicular carcinoma, there are no long-term follow-up studies available to show whether some of these patients may not develop recurrence and/or metastasis after 20–30 years.

It is our opinion that the term "atypical adenoma" can be avoided if careful assessment of a suspicious tumour has failed to show evidence of vascular and/or capsular invasion. The diagnosis of an "atypical adenoma" still worries a lot of surgeons; if malignancy has been virtually ruled out by examination of numerous tissue blocks, diagnosis of a "adenoma" (thus designated as benign) is justified. However, we clearly state in our reports how many blocks were investigated before we arrived at this diagnosis.

Finally, it has to be stressed that currently no modern techniques are available to distinguish between benign and malignant follicular lesions. Neither ultrastructural (Johannessen and Sobrinho-Simoes 1982), nor morphometric (Johannessen and Sobrinho-Simoes 1983; Joensuu et al. 1986) or flow cytometric analysis (Johannessen et al. 1982; Czyz et al. 1994), assessment of nucleolar organiser region-associated proteins (Rüschoff et al. 1994), nor immunohistochemical (Harach et al. 1983; De Micco et al. 1991; Schmid et al. 1994; Czyz et al. 1994; see also the article by Jasani in this issue) or oncogene expression studies (Mizukami et al. 1988; Schmid 1993) have so far proved helpful in the separation of these lesions. Thus to recognise or exclude malignancy still depends entirely on the careful and time-consuming assessment of "old-fashioned" vascular and/or capsular invasion.

Acknowledgement. The authors would like to thank Dr. Thomas Ramsauer for his help.

References

Czyz W, Joensuu H, Pylkkänen L, Klemi PJ (1994) p53 protein, PCNA staining, and DNA content in follicular neoplasms of the thyroid gland. J Pathol 174: 267–274

De Micco C, Ruf J, Chrestian M-A, Gros N, Henry J-F, Carayon P (1991) Immunohistochemical study of thyroid peroxidase in normal, hyperplastic, and neoplastic human thyroid tissues. Cancer 67: 3036–3041

Doniach I (1978) The thyroid gland. In: Symmers WSC (ed) Systemic pathology, vol 4, 2nd edn. Churchill Livingstone, Edinburgh, pp 1976–2037

Evans HL (1984) Follicular neoplasms of the thyroid. Cancer 54: 535–540

Franssila KO, Ackerman LV, Brown CL, Hedinger CE (1985) Follicular carcinoma. Semin Diagn Pathol 2: 101–122

Harach HR, Jasani B, Williams ED (1983) Factor VIII as a marker of endothelial cells in follicular carcinoma of the thyroid. J Clin Pathol 36: 1050–1054

Hazard JB, Kenyon R (1954) The atypical adenoma of the thyroid. Arch Pathol 58: 554–563

Hedinger C, Williams ED, Sobin LH (1988) Histological typing of thyroid tumours 2nd edn. Springer, Berlin Heidelberg New York (International classification of tumours, WHO, no 11)

Hofstädter F (1980) Frequency and morphology of malignant tumours of the thyroid before and after the introduction of iodine-prophylaxis. Virchows Arch [Pathol Anat] 385: 263–270

Hofstädter F, Unterkircher S (1980) Histologische Kriterien zur Prognose der Struma maligna. Pathologe 1: 79–85

Joensuu H, Klemi P, Eerola E (1986) DNA aneuploidy in follicular adenomas of the thyroid gland. Am J Pathol 124: 373–376

Johannessen JV, Sobrinho-Simoes M (1982) Follicular carcinoma of the human thyroid gland. An ultrastructural study with emphasis on scanning electron microscopy. Diagn Histopathol 5: 113–127

Johannessen JV, Sobrinho-Simoes M (1983) Well-differentiated thyroid tumors: problems in diagnosis and understanding. Pathol Annu 18: 255–285

Johannessen JV, Sobrinho-Simoes M, Lindmo T, Tangen KO (1982) The diagnostic value of flow cytometric DNA measurements in selected disorders of the human thyroid. Am J Clin Pathol 77: 20–25

Kahn NF, Perzin KH (1983) Follicular carcinoma of the thyroid: an evaluation of the histologic criteria usid for the diagnosis. Pathol Annu 18: 221–253

Kober F, Wolf G, Depisch D, Galvan G, Keminger K, Ladurner D, Langsteger W, Ogris E, Pimpl W, Roka R, Schmalzer E, Schmid KW, Tuchmann A (1990) Schilddrüsenkarzinom. In: Steindorfer P (ed) Manual der chirurgischen Krebstherapie. Springer, Vienna New York, pp 35–48

Ladurner D, Hofstädter F (1983) Zur Prognose des follikulären Schilddrüsenkarzinoms im Tiroler Strumaendemiegebiet. Langenbecks Arch Chir 360: 267–277

Lang W, Georgii A, Strauch G, Kienzle F (1980) The differentiation of atypical adenomas and encapsulated follicular carcinomas in the thyroid gland. Virchows Arch [Pathol Anat] 385: 125–141

Lang W, Choritz H, Hundeshagen H (1986) Risk factors in follicular thyroid carcinomas. A retrospective followup study covering a 14 year period with emphasis on morphological findings. Am J Surg Pathol 10: 246–255

LiVolsi VA (1990) Follicular lesions of the thyroid. In: Surgical pathology of the thyroid. (Major problems in pathology, vol 22) Sauders, Philadelphia, pp 173–212

Mendelsohn G (1988) Pathology of thyroid disease. In: Mendelsohn G (ed) Diagnosis and pathology of endocrine diseases. Lippincott, Philadelphia, pp 37–137

Mizukami Y, Nonomura A, Hashimoto T, Terahata S, Matsubara F, Michigishi T, Noguchi M (1988) Immunohistochemical demonstration of ras p21 oncogene product in normal, benign, and malignant thyroid tissues. Cancer 61: 873–880

Murray D (1991) The thyroid gland. In: Kovacs K, Asa SL (eds) Functional endocrine pathology, vol 1. Blackwell, Boston, pp 293–374

Rüschoff J, Prasser C, Cortez T, Hohne HM, Hohenberger W, Hofstädter F (1993) Diagnostic value of AgNOR staining in follicular cell neoplasms of the thyroid: comparison of evaluation methods and nucleolar features. Am J Surg Pathol 17: 1281–1288

Schmid KW (1993) Immunohistochemistry and in situ hybridisation in thyroid cancer. Exp Clin Endocrinol 101: 17–22

Schmid KW, Tötsch M, Hittmair A, Feichtinger H, Ladurner D, Hofstädter F (1989) Frequency of medullary thyroid carcinoma in an endemic area. Mod Pathol 2: 90–93

Schmid KW, Greeff M, Hittmair A, Tötsch M, Öfner D, Dockhorn-Dworniczak B, Böcker W, Jasani B (1994) Metallothionein expression in normal, hyperplastic and neoplastic thyroid follicular and parafollicular cells using monoclonal antimetallothionein antibody E9. Endocr Pathol 5: 114–122

Schröder S (1988) Pathologie und Klinik maligner Schillddrüsentumoren. Fischer, Stuttgart

Schröder S, Pfannschmidt N, Dralle H, Arps H, Böcker W (1984) The encapsulated follicular carcinoma of the thyroid. A clinicopathological study of 35 cases. Virchows Arch [A] 402: 259–273

Williams ED (1980) Pathology and natural history. In: Duncan W (ed) Thyroid cancer. Springer, Berlin Heidelbeg New York, pp 47–55

Poorly Differentiated Carcinoma of the Thyroid: An Aggressive Type of Tumour Arising from Thyroid Follicular Epithelium

A. SAKAMOTO

1 Introduction

According to the WHO Histological Classification of Thyroid Tumours (HEDINGER et al. 1988), malignant tumours arising from the follicular epithelium of the thyroid are histologically classified as papillary carcinoma, follicular carcinoma or undifferentiated (anaplastic) carcinoma. The clinical and biological behaviour of papillary and follicular carcinoma are clearly different from that of undifferentiated carcinoma (DONOHUE et al. 1984; FRANSSILA 1973). The first two have a better prognosis, while the latter usually leads to a poor outcome. Both structural and cellular atypia are prominent in undifferentiated carcinoma compared to those in follicular and papillary carcinoma.

The postoperative survival rates of patients with papillary carcinoma versus follicular carcinoma are not significantly different. Most aspects of papillary and follicular carcinomas are similar, though the responses to internal radiotherapy with ^{131}I and the routes of metastases differ between these two types of carcinoma. However, papillary and follicular carcinomas are generally thought to be different types of thyroid cancer.

In this article, the clinicopathological entities of papillary and follicular carcinoma are critically reviewed. Poorly differentiated carcinoma of the thyroid will be discussed as an aggressive type of papillary and follicular carcinoma. Moreover, recent results of investigations into the molecular and genetic levels of poorly differentiated carcinoma will be briefly reviewed.

2 Poorly Differentiated Carcinoma of the Thyroid

Papillary and follicular carcinomas have been considered as separate and independent categories. There seem to be at least two problems with this conventional

Current Topics in Pathology
Volume 91, K.W. Schmid/W. Böcker (Eds.)

histologic classification. The first is that there is no definite difference in prognosis between the two types of carcinoma. Most reports indicate that there is a significant prognostic difference between papillary and follicular carcinomas. Concerning the cancer prognosis, it is not necessary to classify papillary and follicular carcinomas as two different categories.

The second problem is that there are some cases with a poor result even after adequate surgical treatment. Sometimes the poor outcome is apparently caused by anaplastic transformation, but in other cases this type of dedifferentiation does not occur. Among the latter cases, local recurrence sometimes develops, but not all recurrences are fatal. If the recurrence is caused by inappropriate resection of the tumour, the policy regarding extirpation of thyroid tumours should be reconsidered.

Against this background, the present author proposed as long ago as 1983 that "poorly differentiated carcinoma" should be added to the classification of thyroid carcinomas arising from the follicular epithelium (SAKAMOTO et al. 1983). On the basis of histopathological and clinicopathological studies, poorly differentiated carcinoma was designated as an aggressive type of papillary and follicular carcinoma of the thyroid. The histological criteria and biological characteristics are described below.

2.1 Histology

According to our criteria (SAKAMOTO et al. 1983), both papillary and follicular carcinomas consist histologically of glandular and non-glandular components. The glandular components consist of papillary and/or follicular structures, using the terms "papillary" and "follicular" in their descriptive, not their diagnostic sense. Papillary structures present as papillary protrusions into the lumen lined by an intact layer of follicular cells. Follicular structures also show a lumen bounded by an intact cell layer, but without any papillary projections. Non-glandular components included solid, trabecular and scirrhous patterns. The solid pattern shows a sheetlike arrangement of cancer cells. However, squamous metaplasia consisting of cells without cytological features of malignancy does not occur in poorly differentiated carcinoma. The trabecular pattern involves a cord-like arrangement of cancer cells. A few cancer cells are isolated and scattered in the stroma in the scirrhous pattern.

Papillary and follicular carcinomas composed entirely of glandular components except for squamous metaplasia, as described above, are designated "well-differentiated carcinoma". If additional non-glandular components are found in papillary and follicular carcinomas on histological examination, the tumour should be diagnosed as poorly differentiated carcinoma. Therefore there are two types of histological combinations in poorly differentiated carcinoma: either an admixture of glandular and non-glandular components, or a tumour composed exclusively of non-glandular elements.

In poorly differentiated carcinoma, both glandular and non-glandular components are commonly found in the same case. The two components are generally intermingled, not sharply demarcated. In most cases, the glandular component is usually seen in the peripheral area of a tumour, with an irregular border between this component and the surrounding tissues.

2.2 Clinical Characteristics

The incidence of poorly differentiated carcinoma has been reported at between 10% and 20% of papillary and follicular carcinomas (TSUMORI et al. 1985). Among 221 papillary and follicular carcinomas we encountered 186 well-differentiated and 35 poorly differentiated carcinomas (SAKAMOTO et al. 1983). The proportions of poorly differentiated carcinoma among papillary and follicular carcinomas were 15.6% and 17.2%, respectively.

The female: male ratio was 2:1 in our study. This was much lower that the ratio in well-differentiated carcinoma (7:1), but higher than that in undifferentiated carcinoma (1:1).

The mean age of patients with poorly differentiated carcinoma was 55.2 years (females 55.2 years and males 55.3 years). These values were between those for well-differentiated (48.3 years) and undifferentiated carcinomas (63.2 years).

2.3 Postoperative Prognosis

According to our data, the 15-year survival rates associated with papillary and follicular carcinomas, including both the well- and the poorly differentiated types, were 81.2% and 70.5%, respectively. However, these differences in survival between papillary and follicular carcinomas were not significant.

The 5-year survival rate for patients with poorly differentiated carcinomas was 65.0%, and that for patients with well-differentiated carcinomas was 95.1%. The difference in survival rates between the two variants was markedly increased at both the 10- and the 15-year point. The survival curves for well-differentiated and poorly differentiated carcinomas were significantly different ($p < 0.01$) both in the whole series and among the patients without extrathyroidal extension.

2.4 Immunohistochemistry

Immunohistochemical studies have compared various types of thyroid tumous, including benign ones, using various antibodies (PAPOTTI et al. 1993; PILOTTI et al. 1994; YAMAMOTO et al. 1992). Molecular and genetic aspects of thyroid carcinomas have also been analysed immunohistochemically.

Thyroglobulin immunoreactivity has been well investigated. Well-differentiated carcinoma shows almost 100% reactivity. However, the positive rate of undifferentiated carcinoma is quite low. Poorly differentiated carcinoma also has a low immunoreactivity (Harach and Franssila 1988).

The reactivity of the oncogene and suppressor oncogene products and growth factors has been intensively analysed in the past few years. Both p53 and c-erb B2 generally show high reactivity in poorly differentiated carcinoma, but are low in well-differentiated carcinoma (Fagin et al. 1993; Dobashi et al. 1993; Donghi et al. 1993). According to our results (Dobashi et al. 1993), there is a significant difference in the percentages of positive nuclear staining for p53 between well-differentiated and poorly differentiated carcinoma ($p < 0.001$). We suggested that overexpression of p53 does not participate in the process of oncogenesis itself, but is closely related to development of the biologically aggressive subtypes of thyroid carcinoma, poorly differentiated carcinoma and undifferentiated carcinoma.

bcl-2 has been reported as a differentiation-associated marker among thyroid carcinomas. According to Pilotti's data (Pilotti et al. 1994b), the restriction of bcl-2 expression in poorly differentiated and well-differentiated carcinomas was in 84.2% and 13.6% of cases, respectively. They indicated that evaluation of bcl-2 expression can usually be applied to the differentiation of poorly differentiated carcinoma from undifferentiated carcinoma.

Other characterizations show a significant association among specific genetic alterations and histological types. Thus, mutations of the *ras* gene family can be detected in both follicular carcinomas and adenomas (Oyama et al. 1995). Further analysis at molecular and genetic levels should be meaningful for possible diagnostic application and investigation of biological characteristics. Along with these studies, we are now investigating tumour progression from normal or benign conditions to well-differentiated carcinoma, from well-differentiated carcinoma to poorly differetiated ones, and from poorly differentiated carcinoma to undifferentiated malignancy (Dobashi et al. 1994).

2.5 Other Histological Subtypes of Thyroid Cancer Proposed as an Aggressive Variant

Before our proposal of poorly differentiated carcinoma of the thyroid, the EORTC Thyroid Cancer Co-operative Group used the term "less well differentiated carcinoma" (Byar et al. 1979). However, the prognosis of this type of carcinoma did not significantly differ from the conventional types of papillary and follicular carcinomas. Then, after poorly differentiated carcinoma was described as an intermediate category between well-differentiated and undifferentiated carcinomas, various similar disease entities were reported.

The idea of poorly differentiated (insular) carcinoma was derived from the so-called "wuchernde Struma Langhans" (Carcangiu et al. 1984). The term "insular carcinoma" has been commonly used, and its aggressiveness was supported by other authors (Ashfag et al. 1994; Flynn et al. 1988). Both Sakamoto's "poorly differentiated carcinoma" and Carcangiu's "insular carcinoma" can be applied as terms when diagnosing these tumours. However, there are some differences concerning the histological criteria. Some cases of typical insular carcinoma that are completely composed of cribriform-like components must not be classified as poorly differentiated but as well-differentiated carcinoma by Sakamoto's criteria, because of the definite absence of a glandular component in the tumour histology.

"Columnar-cell carcinoma" (EVANS 1986; SOBRINHO-SIMOES et al. 1988) and "tall-cell variant" (JOHNSON et al. 1988) have also proposed as aggressive variants of papillary carcinoma. If columnar-cell carcinoma or the tall-cell variant shows classical papillary structure alone on histology, this may be diagnosed as well-differentiated carcinoma, but not as poorly differentiated by both Sakamoto's and Carcangiu's criteria.

Throughout these variants, the histological criteria differ from one another, although the prognostic features are quite similar, presenting a new problem in the histological classification of thyroid cancer. Further investigation and discussion are needed to establish this type of carcinoma as a disease entity.

References

Ashfag R, Vuitch F, Delgado R, Albores-Saavedra J (1994) Papillary and follicular thyroid carcinomas with an insular component. Cancer 73: 416–423

Byar DP, Green SB, Dor P (1979) A prognostic index for thyroid carcinoma: a study of the EORTC Thyroid Cancer Co-operative Group. Eur J Cancer 15: 1033–1041

Carcangiu ML, Zampi G, Rosai J (1984) Poorly differentiated (insular) thyroid carcinoma: a reinterpretation of Langerhans' "wuchernde Struma". Am J Surg Pathol 8: 665–668

Dobashi Y, Sakamoto A, Sugimura H, Mernyei M, Mori M, Oyama T, Machinami R (1993) Overexpression of p53 as a possible prognostic factor in human thyroid carcinomas. Am J Surg Pathol 17: 375–381

Dobashi Y, Sugimura H, Sakamoto A, Mernyei M, Mori M, Oyama T, Machinami R (1994) Stepwise participation of p53 gene mutation during dedifferentiation of human thyroid carcinomas. Diagn Mol Pathol 3: 1–14

Donghi R, Longoni A, Pilotti S, Michieli P, Della Porta G, Pierotti MA (1993) p53 mutations are restricted to poorly differentiated and undifferentiated carcinomas of the thyroid gland. J Clin Invest 91: 1753–1760

Donohue JH, Goldfien SD, Miller TR (1984) Do the prognoses of papillary and follicular carcinomas differ? Am J Surg 148: 168–173

Evans HL (1986) Columnar-cell carcinoma of the thyroid. A report of two cases of an aggressive variant of thyroid carcinoma. Am J Clin Pathol 85: 77–80

Fagin JA, Matsuo K, Kamakar A, Chen DL, Tang SH, Koeffler HP (1993) High prevalence of mutations of the p53 gene in poorly differentiated human thyroid carcinomas. J Clin Invest 91: 179–184

Flynn SD, Forman BH, Stewart AP (1988) Poorly differentiated (insular) carcinoma of the thyroid: an aggressive subset of differentiated thyroid neoplasms. Surgery 104: 963–970

Franssila KO (1973) Is the differentiation between papillary and follicular thyroid carcinoma valid? Cancer 32: 853–864

Harach HR, Franssila KO (1988) Thyroglobulin immunostaining in follicular thyroid carcinoma: relationship to the degree of differentiation and cell type. Histopathology 13: 43–54

Hedinger C, Williams ED, Sobin LH (1988) Histological typing of thyroid tumours, 2nd edn. Springer, Berlin Heidelberg New York

Johnson TL, Lloyd RV, Thompson NW, Beierwaltes WH, Sisson JC (1988) Prognostic implications of the tall cell variant of papillary thyroid carcinoma. Am J Surg Pathol 12: 22–27

Oyama T, Suzuki T, Hara F, Iino Y, Ishida T, Sakamoto A, Nakajima T (1995) N-ras mutation of thyroid tumor with special reference to follicular type. Pathol Int 45: 45–50

Papotti M, Micca FB, Favero A, Palestini N, Bussolati G (1993) Poorly differentiated thyroid carcinomas with primordial cell component. Am J Surg Pathol 17: 291–301

Pilotti S, Collini P, Del Bo R, Cattoretti G, Pierotti MA, Rilke F (1994a) A novel panel of antibodies that segregates immunocytochemically poorly differentiated carcinoma from undifferentiated carcinoma of the thyroid gland. Am J Surg Pathol 18: 1054–1064

Pilotti S, Collini P, Rilke F, Cattoretti G, Del Bo R, Pierotti MA (1994b) bcl-2 protein expression in carcinomas originating from the follicular epithelium of the thyroid gland. J Pathol 172: 337–342

Rosai J, Carcangiu ML, DeLellis RA (1993) Tumors of the thyroid gland, 3rd series. AFIP, Washington

Sakamoto A, Kasai N, Sugano H (1983) Poorly differentiated carcinoma of the thyroid. A clinicopathologic entity for a high-risk group of papillary and follicular carcinomas. Cancer 52: 1849–1855

Sobrinho-Simoes M, Nesland JM, Johannessen JV (1988) Columnar-cell carcinoma. Another variant of poorly differentiated carcinoma of the thyroid. Am J Clin Pathol 89: 264–267

Tsumori T, Nakao K, Miyata M (1985) Clinico-pathologic study of thyroid carcinoma infiltrating the trachea. Cancer 56: 2843–2848

Yamamoto Y, Izumi K, Otsuka H (1992) An immunohistochemical study of epithelial membrane antigen, cytokeratin and vimentin in papillary thyroid carcinoma. Recognition of lethal and favorable prognostic types. Cancer 70: 2326–2333

Surgical Strategies in Papillary Thyroid Carcinoma

O. GIMM and H. DRALLE

1 Introduction

Papillary thyroid carcinoma is the most common type of thyroid cancer, but its regional occurrence and percentage it makes up of all thyroid malignancies vary greatly. Factors suggested to have an influence are iodine deficiency (MAZZAFERRI 1977; HEITZ et al. 1976), chronic TSH stimulation (SCHOTTENFELD 1985; RICCABONA 1987), radiation (SCHULTZ 1980; CONNARD 1977), genetic factors (OZAKI et al. 1983; STOFFER et al. 1986) and others. The prognosis of patients suffering from papillary thyroid carcinoma is generally considered to be good, 10-year survival rates of more than 80% have been reported (TUBIANA et al. 1985; WOOLNER 1971).

Although surgery is generally regarded as the treatment of choice in papillary thyroid carcinoma, the appropriate extent of surgical resection of both thyroid gland and locoregional lymph nodes is still debated. Some centres recommend total thyroidectomy (BEIERWALTES et al. 1982; MASSIN et al. 1984; VARMA et al. 1970); others report conclusive results after different kinds of subtotal thyroidectomy (CADY et al. 1976; FARRAR et al. 1980; TOLLEFSEN et al. 1972). With regard to locoregional lymph node metastases, their influence on recurrence and in particular on survival has not been proven (CADY et al. 1979; MAZZAFERRI

Current Topics in Pathology
Volume 91, K.W. Schmid/W. Böcker (Eds.)

and Young 1981; Franssila 1975; Rossi et al. 1986; Harwood et al. 1978; McGregor et al. 1985). For this reason, the extent of lymph node surgery at first operation in particular is still controversial (Tollefsen et al. 1964; Block and Miller 1961; Marchetta et al. 1970; McGregor et al. 1985; Sisson and Feldman 1980).

This chapter aims to present our current surgical strategy for patients suffering from papillary thyroid carcinoma, with particular reference to the surgical technique of systematic, compartment-oriented microdissection of locoregional lymph node metastases, recently described for medullary thyroid carcinoma (Dralle et al. 1992).

1.1 Surgery of the Thyroid Gland

Total thyroidectomy has not been described as the treatment of choice in all previous studies. Because of the natural course of papillary thyroid carcinoma – generally good prognosis, a long recurrence-free interval – and the higher morbidity after total thyroidectomy reported in some studies, several authors prefer a more conservative management, i.e. subtotal thyroidectomy (Cohn et al. 1984; DeGroot et al. 1990; Grant and Hay 1988).

In contrast, others recommend total thyroidectomy as the treatment of choice at initial therapy (Clark 1982; Varma et al. 1970). The reasons for total thyroidectomy are:

1. Papillary thyroid carcinoma is often multifocal, whether unilateral or bilateral (Clark et al. 1959). Because of the lack of accurate preoperative diagnostic methods by which to determine multifocality, total thyroidectomy is the only way to remove as much as possible and as much as is necessary of the entire thyroid tumour mass.
2. In patients reoperated on to remove a thyroid remnant, a higher rate of complications after the second operation than after the initial surgery has been described (Bay et al. 1988; Beahrs and Vandertoll 1963).
3. Total thyroidectomy allows postoperative diagnostic measurement of thyreoglobulin (Schlumberger et al. 1981) and treatment with radioiodine (Roesler 1987).

1.2 Surgery of Lymph Nodes

Locoregional lymph node metastasis of malignant tumours is generally considered to worsen the prognosis, and it has been shown that extensive resection can improve the outcome of those patients (Koyama et al. 1985; Siewert et al. 1986). However, in patients with papillary thyroid carcinoma the significance of lymph node metastases is still unclear; some authors have observed survival to be not significantly poorer in patients with lymph node metastases of papillary thyroid carcinoma (McConahey et al. 1986; DeGrot et al. 1990), or have even observed a better outcome in patients with lymph node involvement (Rossi et al. 1986). Therefore, the extent of surgical therapy remains disputed. Some authors recommend selective resection only for grossly involved lymph nodes (Cady 1981); others perform a modified neck dissection (Harwood et al. 1978) or prefer prophylactic lymph node dissection (Ozaki et al. 1988).

We studied the outcome of patients with and without lymph node metastases as well as the influence of different surgical methods of lymphadenectomy, with particular reference to systematic, compartment-oriented microdissection, as recently described for medullary thyroid carcinoma (Dralle et al. 1992).

2 Patients and Methods

We analyzed the data of 342 patients with papillary thyroid carcinoma, out of 728 patients with thyroid cancer operated on at the Medical School of Hanover from 1972 to 1992. Histological diagnosis of papillary thyroid carcinoma was according to the World Health Organization (WHO) typing of thyroid tumours (Hedinger et al. 1988), and staging of primary tumours was done according to the TNM classification for malignant tumours of the UICC (Hermanek and Sobin 1987). Statistical analysis was performed using descriptive tools such as frequency tables and cross tables. Life tables were computed using the product limit estimate introduced by Kaplan and Meier (Kaplan and Meier 1958). Multivariate analysis was done by means of the proportional hazard model of Cox (Cox and Oakes 1984).

2.1 Technique of Systematic, Compartment-Oriented Microdissection of Cervicomediastinal Lymph Nodes

In contrast to the various forms of selective lymphadenectomy (i.e. removal of one or more macroscopically tumour-involved lymph nodes with or without interstitial adipose tissue), the principle of systematic, compartment-oriented microdissection is anatomical en-bloc microdissection of the described compartments below, with their enclosed lymph nodes and adipose and connective tissue, by the aid of magnifying glasses and bipolar coagulation forceps. The sternocleidoid muscle, internal jugular vein, transverse cervical artery, thoracic duct, accessory nerve, brachial plexus, sympathetic trunk and phrenic nerve are identified and preserved.

2.2 Definition of Cervicomediastinal Lymph Node Compartments

Based on the embryological development and the surgical anatomy of the cervicomediastinal lymph node system (Fisch and Sigel 1964; Jackson et al.

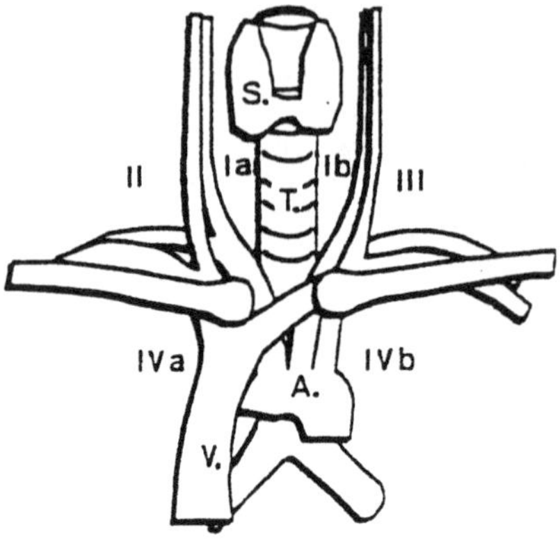

Fig. 1. Hanover compartment classification of regional lymph nodes in the neck and upper mediastinum. *S.*, Thyroid gland; *T.*, trachea; *A.*, aorta; *V.*, superior vena cava

1963), four regional lymph node compartments have been defined (Fig. 1) (DRALLE et al. 1992):

Compartment 1: Cervicocentral lymph node system, right (Ia) and left (Ib) from the trachea, between the trachea and the carotid sheath, and from the hyoid bone down to the brachiocephalic vein, including the submandibular lymph nodes.

Compartments 2 and 3: right (II) and left (III) cervicolateral lymph node system between the carotid sheath and trapezoid muscle, from the subclavian vein up to the hypoglossic nerve, anterior to, posterior to, and between the fascicles of the cervical plexus.

Compartment 4: Mediastinal lymph node system on both sides of the trachea (right IVa, left IVb), from the brachiocephalic vein down to the trachial bifurcation within the anterior and posterior part of the mediastinum.

3 Results

3.1 Age, Sex and pTNM Distribution

From 1972 to 1986 141 patients (101 females, 40 males) with papillary thyroid carcinoma underwent selective lymphadenectomy. The mean age was 47.9 years (range 13.6–82.3 years). The pT categories (UICC) were as follows: pT1 $n = 12$, pT2 $n = 59$, pT3 $n = 19$ and pT4 $n = 51$. In 33 out of 141 patients (23.4%) no lymph node metastases were found; in 108 patients (76.6%) lymph nodes were involved. Distant metastases were diagnosed in 12 patients (8.5%).

Since 1986 60 patients (44 females, 16 males) have undergone systematic lymphadenectomy. Their mean age was 44.2 years (range 12.8–83.5 years). The pT categories were as follows: pT1 $n = 8$, pT2 $n = 26$, pT3 $n = 11$ and pT4 $n = 15$. In 8 out of 60 patients (13.3%) no lymph node metastases were found; in 52 patients (86.7%) lymph nodes were involved. Distant metastases were diagnosed in 5 pa-

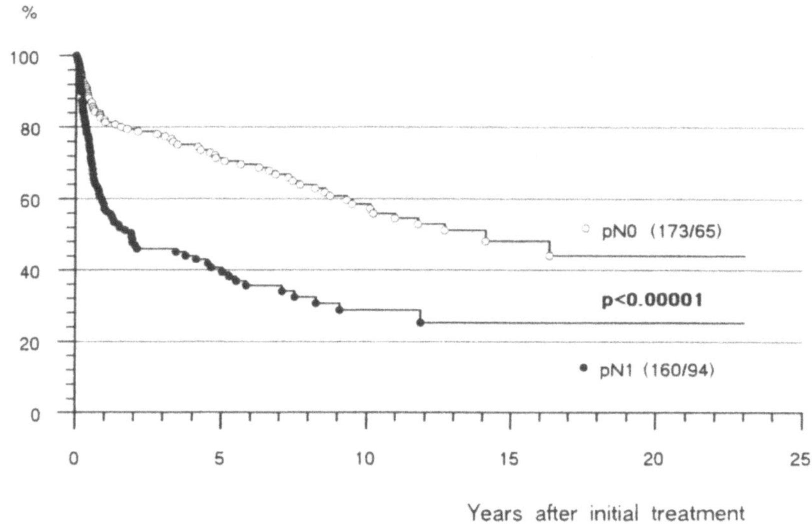

Fig. 2. Cumulative disease-free survival in patients with papillary thyroid carcinoma plotted by initial pN category; pT1–4 tumours

tients (8.3%). Comparing these descriptive features, there was no significant difference between patients who underwent selective surgery and those who had systematic resection. After selective lymphadenectomy we found a mean of 2.2 (range 0–7) tumour-involved lymph nodes out of a mean of 3.9 (range 1–8) resected, whereas after systematic lymphadenectomy a mean of 6.4 (range 0–21) lymph nodes out of a mean of 24.4 (range 4–50) dissected were histologically proven to be involved ($p < 0.001$).

3.2 Recurrence and Survival in Patients With (pN1) and Without (pN0) Lymph Node Metastases

Cumulative disease-free survival in patients with pT1-4 tumours is shown in Fig. 2. The rate of recurrence was much higher in patients with lymph node metastases than in those without ($p < 0.00001$). Because of the high percentage of tumour-positive nodes in patients with pT4 tumour (Fig. 3), one might expect a high influence of lymph node metastases on recurrence in patients with pT4 tumour. Figure 4 shows, however, that we could not verify this assumption. While lymph node metastases had a significant influence on recurrence within the first few years after initial therapy, this influence became insignificant 10 or more years after initial therapy. However, in contrast to what was seen in patients with pT4 tumour, we observed a significant influence of lymph node metastases on recurrence in patients with pT1–3 tumours (Fig. 5, $p < 0.00001$). Much more importantly, we found almost the same results when analysing the influence of lymph node

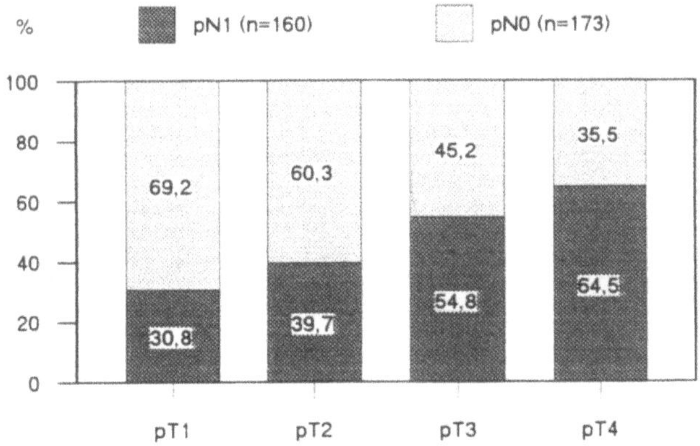

Fig. 3. Distribution of pN categories according to pT category

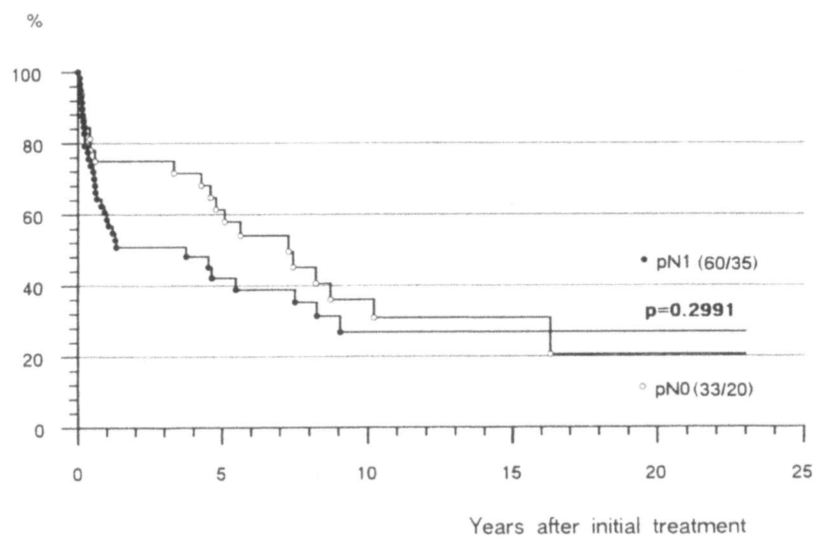

Fig. 4. Cumulative disease-free survival in patients with papillary thyroid carcinoma plotted by initial pN category; pT4 tumours

metastases on survival. Patients with lymph node metastases had a significantly poorer survival than patients without lymph node involvement (Fig. 6, $p < 0.00001$). This influence remained significant when patients with pT1-3 tumours were analysed ($p = 0.001$, Fig. 7), while for those with pT4 tumours no significant influence of lymph node involvement on survival could be found (Fig. 8).

The independent influence of lymph node metastases on recurrence and survival has been shown in various subgroups (SCHEUMANN et al. 1994). Using multivariate analysis, the influence of lymph node metastases on recurrence (risk factor 2.4, $p < 0.00001$) and on survival (risk factor 4.7, $p < 0.00001$) could be verified.

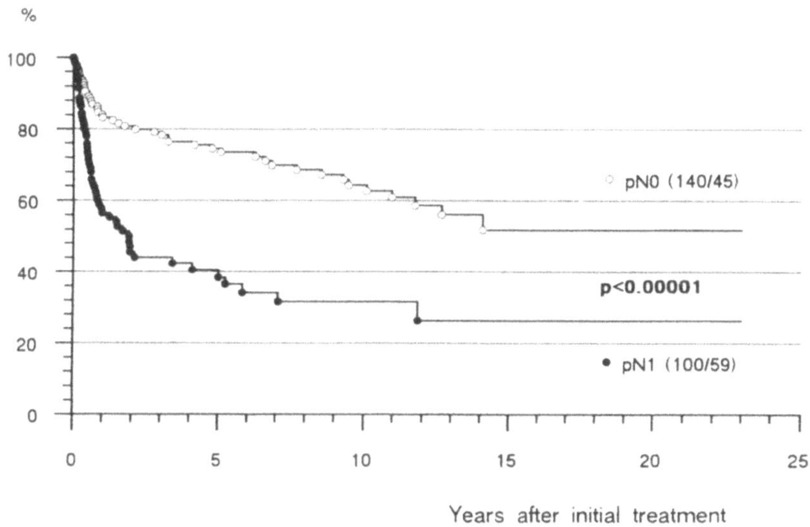

Fig. 5. Cumulative disease-free survival in patients with papillary thyroid carcinoma plotted by initial pN category; pT1–3 tumours

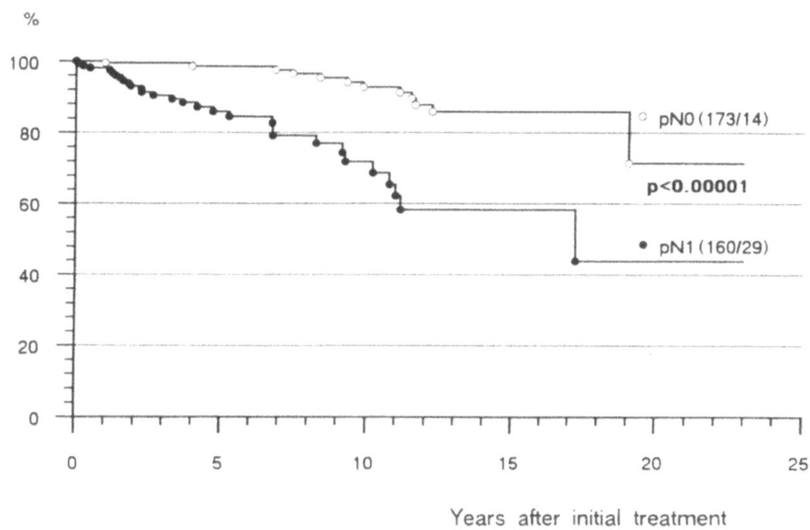

Fig. 6. Cumulative survival of patients with papillary thyroid carcinoma plotted by initial pN category; pT1–4 tumours

3.3 Systematic, Compartment-Oriented Microdissection in Papillary Thyroid Carcinoma

Having shown that lymph node metastases in patients suffering from papillary thyroid carcinoma influence not only the rate of recurrence but also the rate of

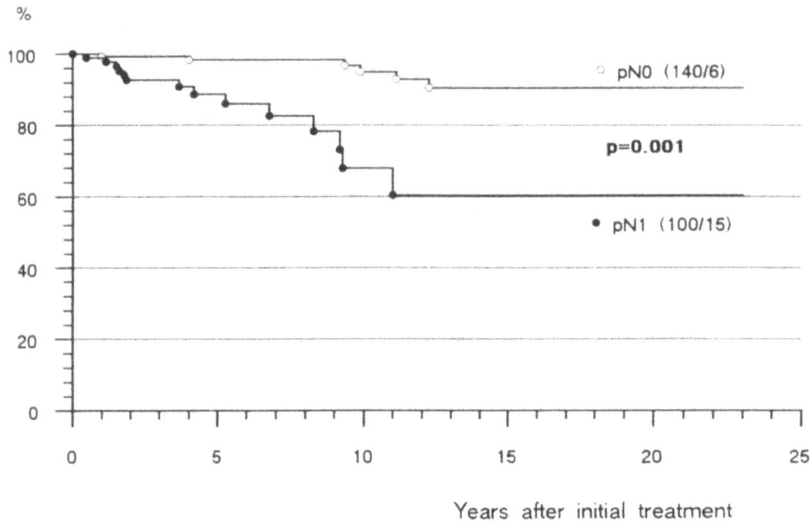

Fig. 7. Cumulative survival of patients with papillary thyroid carcinoma plotted by initial pN category; pT1–3 tumours

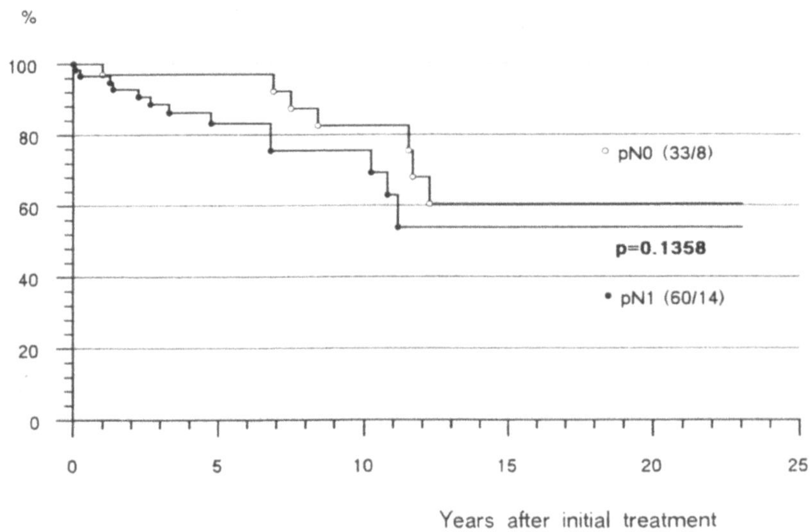

Fig. 8. Cumulative survival of patients with papillary thyroid carcinoma plotted by initial pN category; pT4 tumours

survival, we analysed the influence of the surgical technique on this prognostic factor.

Since 1986 60 patients have undergone systematic lymphadenectomy of the central compartment (C1): 29 patients at initial therapy at the Medical School of

Hanover, 31 patients within 4 weeks after initial therapy performed elsewhere. Systematic lymphadenectomy of the lateral (C2/3) or mediastinal (C4) compartment was performed where there was suspected or proven involvement of lymph nodes. This stage-adapted mode of therapy is worthwhile, because we found histologically proven tumour involvement of lymph nodes of the central compartment (C1) in 72% of cases (Fig. 9), and proven involvement of lymph nodes of the lateral compartment (C2/3) in 28%.

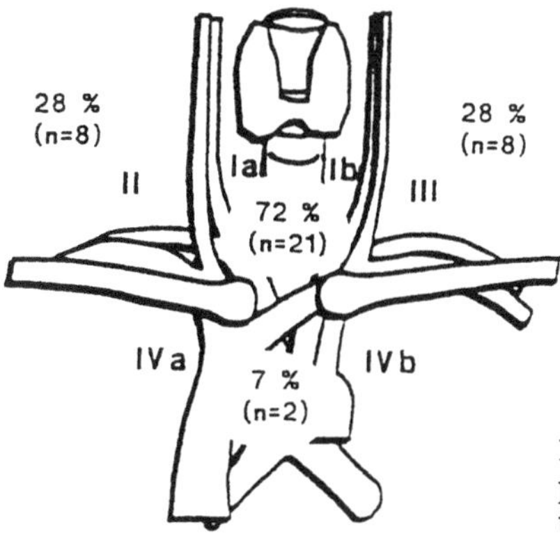

Fig. 9. Percentages of lymph node involvement in 29 patients with papillary thyroid carcinoma at initial therapy at the Medical School of Hanover

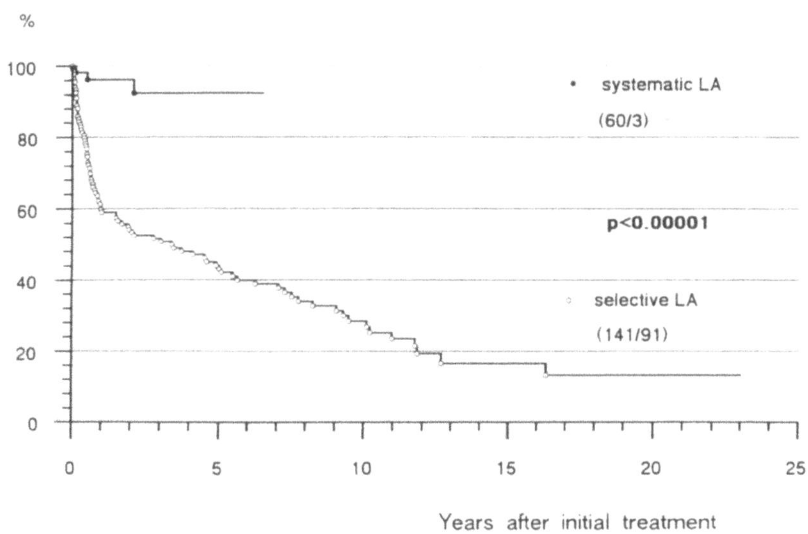

Fig. 10. Cumulative disease-free survival in patients with papillary thyroid carcinoma, plotted by method of lymphadenectomy; pT1–4 tumours. *LA*, Lymphadenectomy

3.4 Results of Systematic, Compartment-Oriented Microdissection in Papillary Thyroid Carcinoma

Cumulative rates of recurrence and survival plotted according to the method of lymphadenectomy performed in patients with pT1-4 tumours are shown in Figs. 10 and 11. The 60 patients who underwent systematic lymphadenectomy had a significantly lower rate of recurrence and a significant higher rate of survival. Three out of 60 patients who underwent systematic lymphadenectomy suffered tumour recurrence and underwent reoperation, and another 3 patients died after systematic lymphadenectomy. All these 6 patients had a pT4 tumor at initial operation and radical surgery was not possible. Figures 12 and 13 show cumulative rates of recurrence and survival among patients with pT1-3 tumours plotted according to the method of lymphadenectomy. The better outcome of patients in whom systematic lymphadenectomy was performed is well shown.

4 Discussion

The influence of locoregional lymph node metastases on recurrence and, in particular, on survival in papillary thyroid carcinoma is still debated (CADY et al. 1979; MAZZAFERRI and YOUNG 1981; FRANSSILA 1975; ROSSI et al. 1986; HARWOOD et al. 1978; MCGREGOR et al. 1985). Especially the extent of lymph node surgery at initial operation is still unclear (TOLLEFESEN et al. 1964; BLOCK and MILLER 1961;

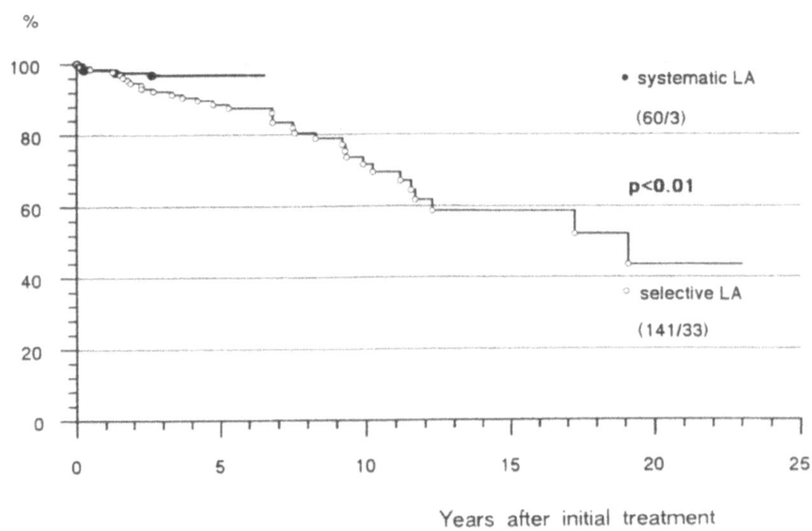

Fig. 11. Cumulative survival of patients with papillary thyroid carcinoma, plotted by method of lymphadenectomy; pT1–4 tumours

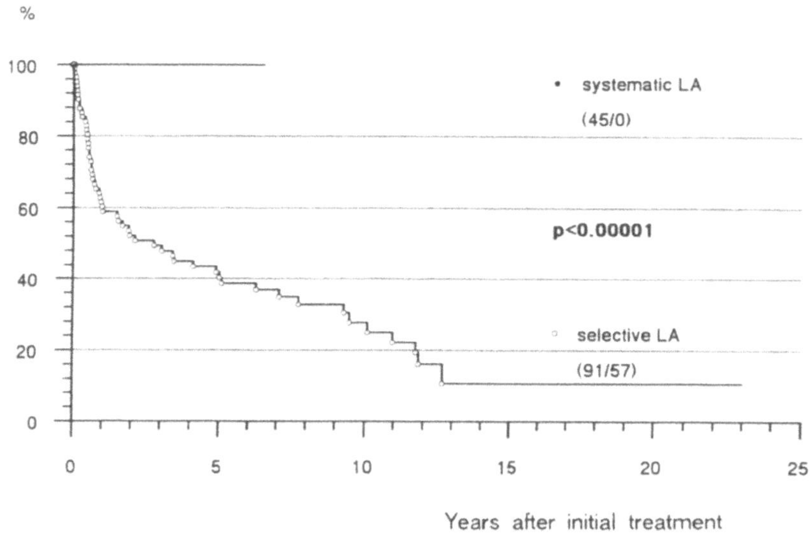

Fig. 12. Cumulative disease-free survival in patients with papillary thyroid carcinoma, plotted by method of lymphadenectomy; pT1–3 tumours.

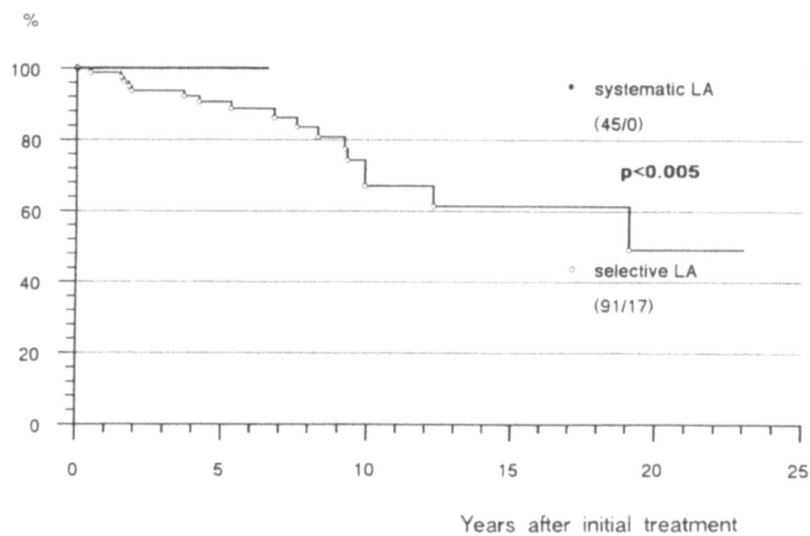

Fig. 13. Cumulative survival of patients with papillary thyroid carcinoma, plotted by method of lymphadenectomy; pT1–3 tumours

MARCHETTA et al. 1970; MCGREGOR et al. 1985; SISSON and FELDMAN 1980). In contrast to many others, we found a significant influence of lymph node metastases on recurrence and on survival using univariate and multivariate analyses. One explanation of this might be that patients treated at the Medical School of

Hanover represent a highly selected patient population with advanced tumour status, extrathyroid tumour extension in a high percentage of cases and extensive lymph node involvement, and therefore our results cannot be applied to all patients with papillary thyroid carcinoma. Another reason might lie in epidemiological or aetiological differences. Patients treated at our clinic come from an area that is iodine-deficient. Thyroid carcinomas that develop in iodine-deficient areas have a different biological behaviour than those arising in iodine-rich areas, typical features being older patient age, a higher proportion of follicular carcinoma, a high incidence of anaplastic thyroid carcinoma, and conversion of longstanding papillary thyroid carcinoma to anaplastic thyroid carcinoma which leads to death. Short mean observation times (MAZZAFERRI and YOUNG 1981), or the classing of papillary and follicular thyroid carcinoma together as differentiated thyroid carcinoma, might be further explanations for the lack of influence of lymph node metastases on survival in papillary thyroid carcinoma found in many other studies.

Having found that lymph node metastases influence the survival of patients with papillary thyroid carcinoma, one should expect a better outcome after removal of all lymph node metastases. Systematic lymphadenectomy seems to be the appropriate technique to remove all lymph node metastases. After selective lymphadenectomy we found a mean of 2.2 (range 0–7) tumour-involved lymph nodes out of a mean of 3.9 (range 1–8) resected. In contrast, after systematic lymphadenectomy a mean of 6.4 (range 0–21) lymph nodes out of 24.4 (range 4–50) dissected were histologically proven to be involved ($p < 0.001$). In our opinion, this is the explanation why patients benefit from systematic lymphadenectomy.

In addition, it has been shown that other therapeutic methods such as radioiodine treatment may fail, especially in micrometastases (SAUTER-BIHL et al. 1991).

5 Conclusions

From our experience, classification of locoregional lymph node compartments, standardization of the surgical technique of compartment-oriented microdissection of cervicomediastinal lymph nodes, and histological evaluation of the exact number of dissected and tumour-involved lymph nodes are essential for a standardized therapy concept. The following conclusions can be drawn from the present data based on our patient series:

- Lymph node metastases are an independent, highly significant prognostic factor in patients suffering from papillary thyroid carcinoma.
- We found tumour involvement of lymph nodes in the central compartment (C1) in 72% of cases; therefore, systematic lymphadenectomy of the central compartment is essential at initial therapy.
- Systematic lymphadenectomy of the lateral (C2/C3) or mediastinal (C4) compartment should be performed in cases where lymph node metastases are suspected or have been proven.

References

Bay V, Engel U, Zornig C (1988) Technik und Komplikationen bei Rezidiveingriffen an der Schilddrüse. Wien Med Wochenschr 100: 352–354

Beahrs O, Vandertoll DJ (1963) Complications of secondary thyroidectomy. Surg Gynecol Obstet 117: 535–540

Beierwaltes WH, Nishiyama RH, Thompson NW, Copp JE, Kubo A (1982) Survival time and cure in papillary and follicular thyroid carcinoma with distant metastases: statistics following University of Michigan therapy. J Nucl Med 23: 561–568

Block MA, Miller JM (1961) Modified neck dissection for thyroid carcinoma. Am J Surg 101: 349–354

Cady B (1981) Surgery of thyroid cancer. World J Surg 5: 3–14

Cady B, Sedgwick CE, Meissner WA, Bookwalter JR, Romagosa V, Weber J (1976) Changing clinical, pathologic, therapeutic and survival patterns in differentiated thyroid carcinoma. Ann Surg 184: 541–553

Cady B, Sedgwick CE, Meissner WA, Wool MS, Salzman FA, Werber J (1979) Risk factor analysis in differentiated thyroid cancer. Cancer 43:810–820

Clark OH (1982) Total thyroidectomy: the treatment of choice for patients with differentiated thyroid cancer. Ann Surg 196: 361–370

Clark RL, White C, Russel EO (1959) Total thyroidectomy for cancer of the thyroid: significance of intraglandular dissemination. Ann Surg 149: 858–866

Cohn KJ, Baeckdahl M, Forsslund G, Auer G, Zetterberg A, Lundell G, Grandberg PO, Loewhagen T, Willems JS, Cade B (1984) Bilogic considerations and operative strategy in papillary thyroid carcinoma: arguments against the routine performence of total thyroidectomy. Surgery 96: 957–970

Connard RA (1977) Summary of thyroid findings in Marshallese 22 years after exposure to radioactive fallout. In: DeGroot LJ (ed) Radiation-associated thyroid carcinoma. Grune and Stratton, New York, pp 241–257

Cox DR, Oakes D (1984) Analysis of survival time data. Chapman and Hall, London

DeGroot LJ, Kaplan EL, McCormick M, Straus FH (1990) Natural history, treatment, and course of papillary thyroid carcinoma. J Clin Endocrinol Metab 71: 414–424

Dralle H, Scheumann GF, Kotzerke J, Brabant EG (1992) Surgical management of MEN 2. Recent Results Cancer Res 125: 167–195

Farrar WB, Cooperman M, James AG (1980) Surgical management of papillary and follicular carcinoma of the thyroid. Ann Surg 192: 701–704

Fisch UP, Sigel ME (1964) Cervical lymphatic system as visualized by lymphography. Ann Otol Rhinol Laryngol 73: 869–882

Franssila KO (1975) Prognosis in thyroid carcinoma. Cancer 36: 1138–1146

Grant CS, Hay D (1988) Local recurrence of papillary thyroid carcinoma after unilateral or bilateral thyroidectomy. Wien Med Wochenschr 100: 342–346

Harwood J, Clark OH, Dunphy JE (1978) Significance of lymph node metastases in differentiated thyroid cancer. Am J Surg 136: 107–110

Hedinger C, Williams ED, Sobin LH (1988) Histological typing of thyroid tumours. 2nd edn. World Health Organization, Geneva, pp 3–11

Hetiz P, Moser H, Staub JJ (1976) Thyroid cancer: a study of 573 thyroid tumors and 161 autopsy cases observed over a thirty-year period. Cancer 37: 2329–2337

Hermanek P, Sobin LH (1987) TNM classification of malignant tumors, 4th edn. Springer, Berlin Heidelberg New York, pp 35–37

Jackson L, Wallace S, Fabr SN, Parke WW, Toy F (1963) Cervical lymphograpy. Laryngoscope 73: 926–941

Kaplan EL, Meier P (1958) Nonparametric estimation from incomplete observation. J Am Statist Assoc 53: 457–481

Koyama Y, Moriya Y, Hojo K (1985) Effects of extended systematic lymphadenectomy for adenocarcinoma of the rectum – significant improvement of survival rate and decrease of local recurrence. Jpn J Clin Oncol 14: 623–632

Marchetta FC, Sako K, Matsuura H (1970) Modified neck dissection for carcinoma of the thyroid gland. Am J Surg 120: 452–455

Massin JO, Savoie JC, Garnier H, Guiraudon G, Leger FA, Bacourt F (1984) Pulmonary metastases in differentiated thyroid carcinoma. Cancer 53: 982–992

Mazzaferri EL (1977) Papillary thyroid carcinoma: the impact of therapy in 576 patients. Medicine (Baltimore) 56: 171–196

Mazzaferri EL, Young RL (1981) Papillary thyroid carcinoma: a 10 year follow-up report of the impact of therapy in 576 patients. Am J Med 70: 511–518

McConahey WM, Hay ID, Woolner LB, van Heerden JA, Taylor WF (1986) Papillary thyroid cancer treated at the Mayo Clinic, 1946 through 1970: initial manifestations, pathologic findings, therapy, and outcome. Mayo Clin Proc 61: 978-996

McGregor GI, Luoma A, Jackson SM (1985) Lymph node metastases from well-differentiated thyroid cancer. Am J Surg 149: 610–612

Ozaki O, Ito K, Kobayashi K, Suzuki A, Manabe Y, Hosoda Y (1983) Familial occurrence of differentiated, nonmedullary thyroid carcinoma. World J Surg 12: 565–571

Ozaki O, Ito K, Kobayashi K, Suzuki A, Manabe Y, Hosoda Y (1988) Modified neck dissection in patients with non advanced, differentiated carcinoma of the thyroid. World J Surg 12: 825–829

Riccabona G (1987) Thyroid cancer: its epidemiology, clinical features and treatment. Springer, Berlin Heidelberg New York, pp 6–50

Roesler H (1987) Thyroid suppression and radioiodine treatment for thyroid cancer. Arch Otolaryngol Head Neck Surg 113: 778–779

Rossi RL, Cady B, Silverman ML, Wool MS (1986) Current results of conservative surgery for differentiated thyroid carcinoma. World J Surg 10: 612–622

Sauter-Bihl ML, Herbold G, Heinze HG, Bihl H (1991) Postoperative externe Radiotherapie des differenzierten Schilddrüsenkarzinoms: wann ist eine alleinige Radiojodtherapie unzureichend? Strahlenther Onkol 167: 267–272

Scheumann GF, Gimm O, Wegener G, Dralle H (1994) Prognostic significance and surgical management of locoregional lymph node metastases in papillary thyroid cancer. World J Surg 18: 559–568

Schlumberger M, Fragu P, Parmentier C, Tubiana M (1981) Thyroglobulin assay in the follow-up of patients with differentiated thyroid carcinomas: comparison of its value in patients with or without normal residual tissue. Acta Endocrinol (Copenh) 98: 215–221

Schottenfeld D (1985) Epidemiology, etiology, and pathogenesis of head and neck cancer. In: Chretien PB, Johns ME, Shedd DP, Strong EW, Ward PH (eds) Head and neck cancer, vol 1. Decker, Philadelphia, pp 6–18

Schultz AC (1980) Childhood irradiation and the incidence of thyroid cancer. Minn Med 63: 535–538

Siewert JR, Lange J, Boettcher K, Becker K, Stier A (1986) Lymphadenektomie beim Magencarcinom. Langenbecks Arch Chir 368: 137–148

Sisson GA, Feldman DE (1980) The management of thyroid carcinoma metastatic to the neck and mediastinum. Otolaryngol Clin North Am 13: 119–126

Stoffer SS, van Dyke DL, Bach JV, Szpunar W, Weiss L (1986) Familial papillary carcinoma of the thyroid. Am J Med Genet 25: 775–782

Tollefsen HR, De Cosse JJ, Hutter RP (1964) Papillary carcinoma of the thyroid: a clinical and pathological study of 70 fatal cases. Cancer 17: 1035–1044

Tollefsen HR, Shah JP, Huvos AG (1972) Papillary carcinoma of the thyroid: recurrence in the thyroid gland after initial surgical treatment. Am J Surg 124: 468–472

Tubiana M, Schlumberger M, Rougier P, Laplanche A, Benhamou E, Gardet P, Caillou B, Travagli JP, Parmentier C (1985) Long-term results and prognostic factors in patients with differentiated thyroid carcinoma. Cancer 55: 794–804

Varma VM, Beierwaltes WH, Nofal MM, Nishiyama RH, Coop JE (1970) Treatment of thyroid cancer: death rates after surgery and after surgery followed by sodium iodine I-131. JAMA 214: 1437–1442

Woolner LB (1971) Thyroid carcinoma: pathologic classification with data on prognosis. Semin Nucl Med 1: 481–502

Growth Factors in Thyroid Cells

R. GÄRTNER

1 Introduction

The thyroid gland is one of those organs in adult mammals that respond to chronic stimulation with increased function and hypertrophy of the epithelial cells, and under certain conditions also with cell proliferation (hyperplasia). This is one of the reasons why the thyroid fascinates not only thyroidologists but also cell biologists and pathologists.

The mechanisms involved in controlling the switch from hypertrophy to hyperplasia are not yet clearly explained. From clinical, epidemiological and in vivo experiments it has been proposed that both thyroid hypertrophy and hyperplasia are exclusively regulated by TSH. There are indeed some strong arguments for the hypothesis that TSH, through its second messenger cAMP, is the main regulator of both the specific functions of the thyroid (iodine uptake, thyroid hormone synthesis and secretion) and growth (DUMONT et al. 1991; LEWINSKI et al. 1993b; ROGER and DUMONT 1984; WILLIAMS et al. 1987; WYNFORD-THOMAS et al. 1987). There are, however, some reasons to suppose that there may be indirect pathways in thyroid growth regulation. In vitro, some groups could not demonstrate a direct mitogenic effect of TSH on highly differentiated thyroid cells using follicle segments or intact follicles, although they respond to other growth factors (GÄRTNER 1992; GÄRTNER et al. 1985; KRAIEM et al. 1990; WATANABE et al. 1985; WESTER-MARK et al. 1978). This is in contrast to monolayer culture systems, where TSH accelerates the basal growth rate of dispersed single cells (GÄRTNER et al. 1990; GORETZKI et al. 1986; HOERMANN et al. 1989; ROGER and DUMONT 1984). Furthermore, in serum-free medium TSH stimulates growth only in the presence of insulin or IGF I (DUMONT et al. 1991; EGGO et al. 1989, 1990; WILLIAMS et al. 1987; WYNFORD-THOMAS et al. 1987). In vivo, mice treated with inhibitors of iodine organification show a lag phase of 3–6 days until thyroid follicular cells

Current Topics in Pathology
Volume 91, K.W. Schmid/W. Böcker (Eds.)

grow, and , what is most remarkable, this is after the endothelial cells have started to proliferate (MANY et al. 1984). Furthermore, in rats there is a strong correlation between iodine deficiency and increase in the DNA content of thyroid glands, but no correlation between serum TSH and the DNA content of thyroids (STÜBNER et al. 1987). By contrast, thyroid weight correlates very well with TSH stimulation. In addition, in hypophysectomized rats, and therefore in the absence of TSH, the thyroid cells proliferate in response to iodine deficiency (LEWINSKI 1981; LEWINSKI et al. 1993a).

The rapid changes in thyroid volume observed in clinical practice, e.g. after the beginning of antithyroid drug therapy or TSH suppression, are mainly due to hypertrophy or a shrinking of cell volume, an increase or decrease in blood circulation, and not to cell proliferation or cell death. While these rapid changes are more closely related to TSH, cell proliferation and apoptosis may be more related to stimulatory or inhibitory local growth factors regulating hyperplasia and involution of the thyroid tissue (GÄRTNER and BECHTNER 1990; STÜBNER et al. 1987). The alternative hypothesis therefore is that not only TSH, but more important autocrine, paracrine and juxtacrine growth factors under the control of TSH and iodine are involved in development of goitre (DUMONT et al. 1991; EGGO and SHEPPARD 1994; GÄRTNER 1992; LEWINSKI et al. 1993b). In this chapter we will review current knowledge of the autocrine and paracrine production of local growth factors of thyroid epithelial cells. These growth factors are not specific for thyroid cells, but abundant in all tissues regulating fetal and childhood growth and may also be involved in the initiation, promotion and progression of neoplasms (BOND et al. 1992; BROWNE 1991; CHEIFETZ et al. 1990; CZECH 1989; DE LARCO and TODARO 1978; DERYNCK 1990; FISHER and LAKSHMANAN 1990; GOSPODAROWICZ et al. 1986; HEARN 1991; HERINGTON 1991; ROBERTS and SPORN 1990; ROBERTSON 1991).

The thyroid tissue is mainly composed of thyroid follicles (70%), endothelial cells and vessels (20%), extracellular matrix and fibroblasts (10%). During fetal and childhood development the thyroid tissue grows in parallel to the gain in body weight. It has been calculated that this increase in cell number requires about six to seven cell divisions. During normal circumstances the weight of the thyroid remains constant in adulthood, with a slow decrease in the senium. Within this time, cell turnover is very rare; only about five divisions per cell during adulthood have been calculated (COCLET et al. 1989). For this reason only a few mitotic cells are found in vivo; they may be due to the compensation of cell death and tissue repair (ROGNONI et al. 1987). Even during maximal growth stimulation through the action of antithyroid drugs only 3% of epithelial cells are in mitosis. These in vivo events are in contrast to in vitro studies with monolayer cells, where a three- to five-fold increase in cell number can be seen within a few days. One therefore has to be careful in interpreting in vitro findings and extrapolating from these to the in vivo events. We are only beginning to understand the interaction network of the growth factors known to stimulate or inhibit thyroid cell proliferation, and in vitro effects are sometimes the opposite of in vivo events (DAWSON et al. 1991). It is, however, so far clear that local growth factors play an important role in both physiological and pathological growth of the thyroid (DUMONT et al. 1991; EGGO and SHEPPARD 1994; FRAUMAN and MOSES 1990; GÄRTNER et al. 1990; LEWINSKI et al. 1993b).

2 Insulin-Like Growth Factors

The insulin-like growth factors (IGFs) are a family of structurally related polypeptides which have profound effects on the proliferation and differentiation of a variety of cell types. The IGFs are synthesized in many cell types and regulated by different factors. Growth hormone (GH) regulates most of the circulating IGF-I produced in the liver and fibroblasts (HERINGTON 1991). The IGFs are bound to specific binding proteins, six of which have so far been identified. The role of these binding proteins is not yet fully understood (OOI and HERINGTON 1988). The IGFs and their binding proteins secreted locally are regulated not only by GH and seem to be involved in autocrine as well as paracrine growth regulation (MINUTO et al. 1989; PHILLIPS et al. 1994; WANG et al. 1990).

While IGF-I has specific receptor (type I receptor), it also binds to the insulin receptor and vice versa. IGF-II has a different receptor and does not interact with the insulin receptor, but does bind to the type I receptor. The type I IGF-I receptor consists of a heterotetrameric arrangement (molecular weight 300 000 Da) of two $\alpha\beta$ subunit dimers. The two α subunits contain the IGF-I binding side, whereas the β subunits, which are linked to the α subunits via disulphide bonding, span the cell membrane and possess intrinsic tyrosine kinase activity within the cytoplasmic domain. The type II receptor is structurally and functionally quite different from the insulin and type I IGF-I receptor: it consists of a single glycosylated polypeptide and contains no tyrosine kinase activity. The type II receptor is identical to the cation-independent mannose 6-phosphate (M-6P) receptor. The receptor is primarily extracellular and has only a small cytoplasmic tail. The receptor binds lysosomal enzymes, containing M-6P residues. It seems to be involved in tissue remodelling, is expressed during growth induction and seems per se not to be involved in the mitogenic effect induced by IGF-II (CZECH 1989).

Thyroid cells secrete IGF-I and their binding proteins (IGFBPs), first demonstrated by MAK et al. (1985). Since then IGF-I also been shown to be an autocrine factor in human (OLLIS et al. 1989; ONODA et al. 1992; TODE et al. 1989) sheep (BACHRACH et al. 1988, 1989; EGGO et al. 1990), FRTL5 (MACIEL et al. 1988; TRAMONTANO et al. 1986) and porcine thyroid cells (BEERE et al. 1991; HOFBAUER et al. 1996; RAFFERZEDER et al. 1993). In vitro, IGF-I and insulin are important comitogens along with TSH for thyroid cells; this has been shown in human, dog, sheep, porcine, rat and FRTL5 thyroid cells (BRANDI et al. 1987; EGGO et al. 1984; HOERMANN et al. 1989; MACIEL et al. 1988; ROGER and DUMONT 1984; SMITH et al. 1986; TAKASU et al. 1989; TRAMONTANO et al. 1986; WILLIAMS et al. 1987). IGF-I mRNA expression is stimulated by TSH and forskolin, inhibited by iodine and unchanged by EGF (HOFBAUER et al. 1996). The growth response to TSH under low-iodine conditions is abolished in the presence of a blocking type I IGF receptor antibody (aIR3) (MACIEL et al. 1988; RAFFERZEDER et al. 1993). These results clearly identify IGF-I as an autocrine growth factor for thyroid cells, which is under the control of TSH and iodine.

Although IGF-I seems to be mainly a growth factor, there is now good agreement that it also has a role as a differentiation factor. Along with TSH, IGF-I enhances the thyroid peroxidase and thyroglobulin mRNA, iodine uptake and organification (EGGO et al. 1990) and TSH-stimulated cAMP formation (BRENNER-GATI et al. 1989). The mechanism responsible for the stimulation of thyroglobulin gene expression is the ability of IGF-I (and insulin) to modulate the level of thyroid transcription factor 2 (TTF-2), which then results in increased expression of the thyroglobulin gene (SANTISTEBAN et al. 1992). In immunohistochemical studies both IGF-I and the type I IGF receptor have been demonstrated in thyroid epithelial cells in normal tissue (MINUTO et al. 1989). IGF-I (WILLIAMS et al. 1989) and the type I IGF receptor (VANNELLI et al. 1990) have been shown to be overexpressed in thyroid adenomatous tissue. In addition, IGF-I has been shown to be an autocrine growth factor for human thyroid cells from benign adenomas and for a human thyroid cancer cell line derived from a papillary thyroid cancer (ONODA et al. 1992). It may therefore be concluded that the autocrine IGF-I action in normal tissue, which is regulated via the cAMP-dependent pathway, is autonomously overexpressed in neoplastic tissue, inducing autonomous growth of thyroid epithelial cells. The mechanisms inducing this autonomous IGF-I action are still unknown, but a correlation to mutations in G-proteins is supposed (DUMONT et al. 1991), or this action may be due to the hyperfunctioning mutated TSH receptor in thyroid adenomas (PARMA et al. 1993). In addition, the number of type II IGF/M-6P receptors is higher in thyroid cancer tissues than in adjacent non-neoplastic tissues (YASHIRO et al. 1991), suggesting an important role of this receptor in thyroid neoplasia.

Acromegalic patients have not only thyroid hyperplasia, but in about 60% of their goitres adenomas have been detected. This may imply that not only IGF-I is responsible for mormal hyperplasia, but chronic stimulation with IGF-I may initiate the development of benign adenomas. The incidence of thyroid cancer is not increased in these patients (WUESTER et al. 1991). Thyroid cells express no GH receptors, so the goitrogenic effect of IGF-I may be mediated either by the endocrine pathway or by the paracrine secretion of fibroblasts within the thyroid (BECHTNER et al. 1992), known to respond to GH binding with an IGF-I secretion.

IGF-II is also produced in thyroid cells in culture (EGGO et al. 1990). FRTL5 cells transfected with the sequence of rat IGF-II had a significantly higher basal growth rate, did not respond to IGF-I, but had not lost their ability to respond to TSH (VENEZIANI et al. 1992). A specific receptor antibody bolcking both IGF-I and IGF-II receptor (sm1.2) abolished the basal growth acceleration in these transfected cells, suggesting an autocrine growth stimulation of IGF-II comparable to that of IGF-I.

Thyroid cells also produce and secrete IGF binding proteins (IGFBPs), and it seems that these binding proteins modulate the autocrine IGF actions both positively and negatively (OOI and HERINGTON 1988; WANG et al. 1990). In contrast to IGF-I, the secretion of IGFBP from sheep thyroid cells is inhibited by TSH and cortisol (BACHRACH et al. 1991; PHILLIPS et al. 1994) and stimulated by EGF and phorbol esters (EGGO et al. 1990). Mainly IGFB-2, -4 and -5 could be identified, but no IGFBP-1 or -6, in ovine thyroid cell culture (PHILLIPS et al. 1994). In FRTL5 cells a biphasic effect of IGFBP-1 on IGF-I action is described (FRAUMAN and MOSES 1990). Low concentrations enhance the effect of IGF-I, whereas higher concentrations inhibit the IGF-I action. As the affinity of IGF-I to the IGFBP is comparable to the affinity to the type I receptor, it may be hypothesized that IGFBPs compete with the IGF receptors and therefore represent an additional modulatory mechanism of IGF-I action. In serum the IGFBPs prolong the halflife of IGFs. In tissue extracts of papillary cancer the IGF-I content was comparable to that of normal thyroid tissue, whereas the IGFBP activity was significantly increased in papillary cancer tissue (YASHIRO et al. 1994), indicating a possible role of IGFBP in cell proliferation in papillary cancer.

The autocrine action of the IGFs and their binding proteins seems to be a more important factor in thyroid cell proliferation and differentiation than previously supposed. At least in vitro, IGF-I is an important cofactor and modulator of TSH action. Further experiments are necessary to understand the role of the IGFs, their binding proteins and receptor interaction in thyroid cell differentiation and proliferation.

3 Epidermal Growth Factors

The epidermal growth factor (EGF) is now known to be a member of an extended family of growth factors, including the closely related transforming growth factor-α (TGFα) (DERYNCK 1990) and amphiregulin, both of which are produced in several mammalian tissues (BROWNE 1991; FISHER and LAKSHMANAN 1990). Whereas mouse EGF was originally isolated from the submaxillary gland (COHEN 1962), the human EGF was first isolated from the urine of pregnant women (GREGORY 1975). It has been called "urogastrone" because it inhibits gastric juice secretion. The amino acid sequence of EGF is highly conserved and mouse and human EGF are remarkably similar. Of the 53 amino acids (molecular weight 6045 Da), only 16 are different, and the structure (three loops held together by disulphide bonds) is identical. EGF is synthesized and stored in a high molecular weight precursor form (74 000 Da) which is stable between pH 5 and 8. It consists of two molecules [1–53] EGF and two molecules of an arginine esterase protein. At low pH this complex dissociates to release EGF, probably due to this intrinsic enzyme activity. Of special interest is the fact that the EGF precursor can be incorporated into the cell membrane and act as a direct growth stimulator to the neighbouring cell (juxtacrine action) or bind to proteins of the matrix (BROWNE 1991).

Most mammalian cells express an EGF receptor (c-erbB 1), a well characterized member of the tyrosine kinase receptor family (HSUAN et al. 1989). The EGF receptor is a single-chain glycoprotein which comprises an extracellular binding domain, a small transmembrane domain and a C-terminal intracellular tail with a protein kinase domain and three autophosphorylation sites (tyrosine, serine and threonine). Binding of EGF to the receptor is followed by an increase in the phophorylation of a number of intracellular regulatory key proteins such as phospholipases, protein kinases and other regulatory proteins. The EGF-receptor complex is rapidly internalized and degraded. Ligand binding to the EGF receptor is followed by receptor autophosphorylation and followed by the augmentation of many phosphorylation processes in the thyroid cell, and, in some cells, activation of the phosphatidylinositol cascade (RASPE et al. 1989). The proto-oncogene *c-myc* is also enhanced as an very early event after EGF stimulation (HELDIN and WESTERMARK 1988).

TGFα has a similar primary structure to EGF (DERYNCK 1990), is produced from a similar precursor, and binds to and activates the same receptor. TGFα is also assumed to act as a paracrine, autocrine and juxtacrine growth factor. Most of the in vitro experiments have been performed with EGF because it has been easily available before TGFα. As TGFα and EGF share the same receptor it could be that many effects attributed to EGF may be caused by TGFα in vivo. So far, EGF mRNA has been detected in the mouse thyroid, but not in other species. In contrast, TGFα mRNA has been found in human thyroid carcinoma (MIYAMOTO et al. 1989), FRTL5 cells (COLLETTA et al. 1989) and porcine thyroid follicles (GÄRTNER 1992).

As it is for many other cell types, EGF is a very potent growth factor for thyroid cells in vitro (BOURKE et al. 1991; EGGO et al. 1984; GÄRTNER et al. 1985; PRATT et al. 1989; ROGER and DUMONT 1982; WESTERMARK et al. 1983). In intact porcine thyroid follicles, the mitogenic effect of EGF on thyroid cells is inhibited by TSH- or cAMP-activating substances. When EGF and IGF-I are added to the culture medium, the growth response of thyroid epithelial cells exceeds that induced by fetal calf serum and is not only additive but synergistic (GÄRTNER et al. 1990). In porcine thyroid follicle fragments in suspension culture, the number of EGF receptors is increased by TSH stimulation through the adenylate cyclase pathway (WESTERMARK et al. 1986). Therefore it has been supposed that TSH-induced cell proliferation may be also mediated through this pathway. In short-term experiments, however, TSH down-regulates EGF receptor binding in human cells (DI CARLO et al. 1990) and TSH has no effect on EGF binding in sheep thyrocytes (EGGO et al. 1989). In contrast, EGF additive to TSH stimulates thyroid cell mitogenesis in rat organ culture (ZEREK-MELEN et al. 1990). In organ culture, however, paracrine factors derived from cells other than thyrocytes may be activated and responsible for this additive growth promoting effect of TSH and EGF.

In contrast to IGF-I, the action of EGF is followed by a reversible loss of differentiation expression in dog (ROGER and DUMONT 1982) and human (TSENG et al. 1989) thyroid cells. It inhibits iodide uptake and organification not only in vitro, but also in vivo (BLACK et al. 1990) and decreases the TSH-induced cAMP formation (WATERS et al. 1987). In human thyroid cells, both EGF and TGFα suppress the HLA class II expression (TODD et al. 1990).

Whereas in isolated human thyrocytes form normal as well as thyroid tissue from patients with Graves' disease, the EGF receptor is always expressed on the cell surface (MIYAMOTO et al. 1989); this is not the case in vivo. In normal thyroid tissue, EGF and the EGF receptor are not detected or are detected in only a very few epithelial cells using immunohistochemistry techniques. Weak staining was found in two out of eight cases of Graves disease, and in 7 out of 10 follicular adenomas. Stronger expression was found in 100% of follicular and papillary carcinomas (GORGOULIS et al. 1992). In normal thyroid tissue too TGFα was detected only in a very few epithelial cells, whereas it was present in 30% of thyroid adenomas and in 50%–80% of carcinomas. Coexpression of EGF receptor, TGFα and *c-myc* was found in 8 of 19 papillary carcinomas (HAUGEN et al. 1993). It has also been shown that thyroid carcinomas expressing EGF and EGF receptor, or TGFα and EGF receptor, or all three, tend to be associated with lymph mode metastasis. Earlier studies also revealed that high TGFα/EGF and EGF receptor expression are associated with a higher frequency of relapse and lymph node metastasis than absence of the same (AASLAND et al. 1990; KANAMORI et al. 1989; LEMOINE et al. 1991; MAKINEN et al. 1988; SONG 1991). It is of interest that transformed FRTL5 cells that overexpress TGFα do not form tumours in nude mice and are unable to grow in soft agar (COLLETTA et al. 1991). Therefore overexpression of TGFα in thyroid cells is not sufficient to reproduce the transformed phenotype and additional proposed point mutations (i.e. of *ras* oncogene) seem to be necessary for initiating malignancy.

The highest amounts of TGFα expression in different normal human tissues are found in the endothelial cells, respiratory epithelial cells, and the epithelial cells of the gastrointestinal tract and the kidney (YASUI et al. 1992). By contrast, the expression of TGFα in thyroid epithelial cells is very weak. In conclusion, the question of whether both TGFα and /or EGF are expressed in adult normal thyroid epithelial cells is still unanswered. It is also not known whether these closely related growth factors have separate biological effects, e.g. in initiating or promoting neoplasia. In lymphocytic thyroiditis, TGFα (but not EGF) and EGF receptor at both the protein and the mRNA level have been detected in all cases observed (LEMOINE et al. 1991). This confirms the hypothesis that the abnormal TGFα and EGF receptor expression in adults is not restricted to neoplasia.

Tissues from multinodular goitres after surgery have been investigated for their EGF receptor content and compared with the recurrence rate and number of lesions. This study, with more than 300 cases, revealed a good correlation between severity of disease and recurrence rate, with receptor density (SUGENOYA et al. 1992) indicating a possible role of EGF/TGFα in sporadic nodular goitre.

4 Fibroblast Growth Factors

The fibroblast growth factor (FGF) family represents a new class of polypeptide growth factors with biological and structural properties significantly different from those described above. Since the FGFs all bind to heparin, it has been suggested that these growth factors should be classified as heparin-binding growth factors (HBGF; HEARN 1991). This term would better reflect their common structural features and should not mislead one into a restricted interpretation of their biological significance. So far seven members of this family are well known. The first two are acidic and basic FGF (aFGF and bFGF); they have similar tissue distribution and are found in a variety of cells of epithelial, mesenchymal and neural lineage. Further members are the recently characterized keratocyte growth factor (KGF) and four oncogene products (int-2, hst/KS3, FGF 5 and 6; GOSPODAROWICZ et al. 1986; HEARN 1991).

The stability of aFGF and bFGF in vitro and their binding to the receptor are enhanced in the presence of heparin. The receptors belong to the IgG family and exhibit tyrosine kinase activity. The FGFs are potent growth factors for mammalian cells, are chemotactic for fibroblasts and endothelial cells and stimulate the expression of intracellular proteins like actin and ornithine decarboxylase. Angiogenesis seems to be one major biological fuction of the FGFs (Hearn 1991). Thyroid epithelial cell proliferation in vitro is stimulated by both bFGF and aFGF, as has been demonstrated in dog, pig, calf and FRTL5 cells (Black et al. 1990; Emoto et al. 1991; Logan et al. 1992; Pang and Hershman 1990). In human thyroid cells in primary culture, bFGF had no effect on growth, whereas pSV3 neotransfected cells were stimulated to growth (Taylor et al. 1993). In FRTL5 cells, 3H-thymidine incorporation is enhanced by bFGF, but TSH-induced cAMP is reduced and TSH receptor mRNA decreased after bFGF treatment (Pang and Hershman 1990). More importantly, it has been shown that porcine thyroid cells release bFGF into the culture medium (Bechtner et al. 1993; Greil et al. 1989) and express bFGF mRNA (Emoto et al. 1991). It has been demonstrated that isolated thyroid follicles release bFGF into the culture medium. This conditioned medium is able to stimulate fibroblast and endothelial cell proliferation as well as angiogenesis in the chorioallantois membrane assay (Bechtner et al. 1993). The biological activity of the conditioned medium is enhanced when thyroid follicles are stimulated to growth with EGF and decreased by TSH and iodine (Bechtner et al. 1993; Gärtner et al. 1987; Greil et al. 1989). Although bFGF also weakly stimulates thyrocyte proliferation, bFGF seems to be mainly a paracrine rather than an autocrine growth factor, enhancing the concomitant growth of fibroblasts and small vessels during thyroid gland and/or goitre development. This hypothesis is confirmed by the known important role of FGF in angiogenesis (Thomas and Gimenez-Gallego 1986), but has yet to be further elaborated.

In vivo application of recombinant acidic FGF for 6 days induced colloid accumulation in rat thyroids with flat quiescent epithelium but without obvious proliferation (Chanoine et al. 1992; De Vito et al. 1992).

Immunohistochemical studies demonstrate the localization of aFGF and bFGF in the cytoplasm of neoplastic cells, especially in the marginal region of follicular adenoma, follicular carcinoma and papillary carcinoma. In normal thyroids or hyperplastic regions no aFGF or bFGF has been found. This implies an important role of the FGFs in neoplastic proliferation of thyroid epithelial cells rather than in hyperplasia (Kodama et al. 1994).

5 Transforming Growth Factor-β

Transforming growth factor-β (TGFβ) was originally identified as a factor which stimulates colony formation of untransformed rodent cells in soft agar (De Larco and Todaro 1978). Within the last 10 years two forms of TGFβ have been isolated and three further ones identified by screening cDNA libraries. Further similar polypeptides have been identified, belonging to the family of TGFs: inhibin, activin, bone morphogenetic proteins (BMPs), anti-müllerian hormone and a series of further proteins important for development. In vitro, TGFβ is produced in a latent form; the active TGFβ is a homodimer of a molecular weight of 25 kD. The latent form can be transformed in vitro to its active form by acidic treatment or proteolytic cleavage, especially plasmin. Urokinase-like plasminogen activator is secreted by thyroid cells (Cowin and Bidey 1994; Mak et al. 1984) and promotes plasmin generation in the presence of plasminogen (Flaumenhaft et al. 1992). Besides this possible in vivo activation, which may also occur in within the thyroid gland, it has recently been shown that the TGFβ molecule contains a mannose-6-phosphate residue, suggesting that it can bind to the type II IGF/M-6P receptor and can thereby be activated through lysosomal enzyme activity (Purchino et al.). In serum TGFβ is bound to α_2-macroglobulin, an antagonist of its biological activity. Two types of receptors for TGFβ have been identified, which bind both TGFβ_1 and TGFβ_2. The signal transduction of the TGFβ-receptor complex is unknown (Cheifetz et al. 1990; Roberts and Sporn 1990; Robertson 1991). There are multiple biological activities of TGFβ; they include stimulation of the production of integrins, extracellular matrix formation, tissue repair, inflammation and embryogenesis and differentiation processes. In most in vitro experiments, TGFβ inhibits growth of epithelial cells of various origins.

It is obvious that TGFβ is also produced and secreted in the thyroid epithelial cells. TGFβ mRNA has been detected in human thyroid epithelial cell (Grubeck-Loebenstein et al. 1989). It inhibits thyroid cell proliferation as demonstrated in human, porcine, and sheep thyroid cells in primary culture and in FRTL5 cells (Cirafici et al. 1992; Colletta et al. 1989; Cowin et al. 1992; Gärtner et al. 1990; Grubeck-Loebenstein et al. 1989; Moris et al. 1988; Tsushima et al. 1988). In human thyroid primary culture it inhibits both basal and TSH- and EGF-stimulated growth. This growth inhibition is associated with an inhibition of PCNA (proliferating cell nuclear antigen) synthesis. It also completely inhibits the cAMP-induced stimulation of iodine uptake and thyroperoxidase synthesis. Since TSH-induced cAMP generation was not affected by TGFβ while most of the effects of dibutyryl cAMP were inhibited, it is supposed that TGFβ acts at a step distal to cAMP generation (Taton et al. 1993). This is contrast to the effect of TGFβ on FRTL5 cells, where TGFβ inhibits only PKC- but not PKA-mediated DNA synthesis. However, it does inhibit 8-bromo-cAMP-induced iodine uptake (Pang et al. 1992).

It has also been suggested that TGFβ is an important inhibitory growth factor responsible for growth inhibition in thyroid glands with sufficient iodine supplementation, since in nodular goitre lower amounts of TGFβ were found than in Graves' disease (Grubeck-Loebenstein et al. 1989). This is supported by the fact that in sheep thyroid cells, a higher amount of TGFβ mRNA was found when culture medium was supplemented with iodine dosages high enough to inhibit cell proliferation (Yuasa et al. 1992). In human thyroid cells in culture, iodine (10 μmol/l) doubled the mRNA for latent TGFβ_1, but no increase of the active TGFβ was found (Cowin and Bidey 1994). In intact porcine thyroid follicles this could not be confirmed (Gärtner 1992). As TGFβ is also produced by lymphocytes, endothelial cells and fibroblasts, TGFβ bioactivity or mRNA derived from total thyroid tissue may come from these other cells. In rats treated with goitrogens (methimazole) to induce hyperplastic goitres, the TGFβ mRNA increased progressively at 1 and 2 weeks of goitrogen treatment, but decreased during goitre involution, indicating that TGFβ may be involved in temporary stabilization and/or matrix modulation during thyroid hyperplasia (LOGAN et al. 1994). This is confirmed by the fact that in porcine thyroid follicles, TGFβ mRNA expression is significantly increased during EGF stimulation, but not during iodine supplementation (GÄRTNER 1992).

Isolated thyroid cells from normal and neoplastic tissue respond inversely to TGFβ, and SV40 transfected thyroid cells are also not inhibited by TGFβ (DAWSON et al. 1991; WYLLIE et al. 1991). It may therefore be suggested that the lack of responsiveness to TGFβ may be a further factor involved in the mechanism of maintainance or progression of thyroid neoplasia.

6 Other Growth Factors

A series of other, less investigated growth factors have been identified as products of thyroid epithelial cells or have a modulatory effect on thyroid cell growth and function. Like the growth factors described above, *endothelin* is synthesized by many cell types of various lineages. It has been detected in human, porcine and FRTL5 cells (COLIN et al. 1992; TSENG et al. 1993) and different effects of endothelin on growth and function have been described. In human thyroid cell culture, endothelin inhibited thyroglobulin release and had no effect on proliferation (JACKSON et al. 1992). This is in contrast to the findings of others, who observed a growth stimulatory effect on human thyroid cells (EUGUCHI et al. 1993). In FRTL5 cells, endothelin stimulated growth synergistically with IGF-I, but reduced the proliferative effect of TSH. Endothelin production and secretion is stimulated by TGFβ in hnman thyroid cells but only synthesized and not released during TSH stimulation (TSENG et al. 1993). Since endothelin is a vasoconstrictor, one may speculated that endothelin is a paracrine growth factor locally regulating thyroid perfusion. Further experiments are necessary to clarify the role of endothelin in thyroid cell autoregulation.

Hepatocyte growth factor (HGF) is a mitogenic factor in different cells, acting through the tyrosine kinase encoded by the *met* proto-oncogene. In dog thyroid cell in primary culture, this HGF exceeds the effect of TSH and EGF on cell proliferation. HGF inhibits TSH- and forskolin-induced iodine uptake. This may explain the important role of *met* oncogene expression in some thyroid tumors (DREMIER et al. 1994).

Platelet-derived growth factor (PDGF) and its receptor could not be found in normal thyroid cells in culture; however, it seems to be an important growth-promoting factor in thyroid cells derived from papillary cancer (HELDIN et al. 1991; USUKI et al. 1989).

Lymphokines have been identified as being produced and secreted in thyroid cells (TOHYAMA et al. 1992), and some of their receptors seem to be expressed on thyrocytes. The role of these lymphokines seems to be paracrine (EGGO and SEPPARD 1994) more than autocrine, but some effects on specific functions of thyroid cells have been described, such as down-regulation of iodine uptake and thyroid hormone release independent of the cAMP pathway (Nolte et al. 1994).

7 Conclusion

Growth factors, mainly from the IGF, EGF, TGFβ and FGF families, together with their receptors, have been identified in thyroid epithelial cells from various species both in vivo in normal tissue and, abundantly, in thyroid adenomatous tissue or neoplasia. While the IGFs seem to be more related to benign and differentiated growth, the EGFs, TGFβ and the FGFs are connected with inflammation and neoplasia, although not exclusively. From the data available it cannot be concluded that growth factors or their receptors are directly involved in initiating neoplasia. Point mutations in oncogenes such as the *ras* oncogenes or others may be more important for initiating neoplasia (Dumont et al. 1991). The growth factors more probably play a role in the maintenance of growth and in paracrine communication with endothelial cells and fibroblasts (Gärtner et al. 1987). Overexpression of growth factors may be the result of initial point mutations of oncogenes and/or G-proteins and necessary concomitant factors for the maintenance and promotion of neoplasia.

References

Aasland R, Akslen LA, Varhaug JE, Lillehaug JR (1990) Co-expression of the genes encoding transforming growth factor-alpha and its receptor in papillary carcinomas of the thyroid. Int J Cancer 46: 382–387

Bachrach LK, Eggo MC, Hintz RL, Burrow GN (1988) Insulin like growth factors in sheep thyroid cells: action, receptors and production. Biochem Biophys Res Commun 154: 861–867

Bachrach LK, Liu FR, Burrow GN, Eggo MC (1989) Characterization of insulin-like growth factor-binding proteins from sheep thyroid cells. Endocrinology 125: 2831–2838

Bachrach LK, Eggo MC, Burrow GN, Liu F, Tram T, Powell DR (1991) Regulation of insulin-like growth factor-binding protein messenger ribonucleic acid levels in sheep thyroid cells. Endocrinology 128: 1967–1973

Bechtner G, Pötscher C, Gärtner R (1992) Role of autocrine and paracrine factors in thyroid follicle growth. Thyroidol Clin Exp 4: 1–5

Bechtner G, Rieder B, Linsenmaier U, Kellermann J, Greil W, Gärtner R (1993) Isolation and partial molecular characterization of basic fibroblast growth factor from isolated porcine thyroid follicles and entire porcine thyroid glands. Acta Endocrinol (Copenh) 129: 458–466

Beere HM, Soden J, Tomlinson S, Bidey SP (1991) Insulin-like growth factor-I production and action in porcine thyroid follicular cells in monolayer: regulation by transforming growth factor-beta. J Endocrinol 130: 3–9

Black EG, Logan A, Davis JRE, Sheppard MC (1990) Basic fibroblast growth factor affects DNA synthesis and cell function and activates multiple signalling pathway in rat thyroid FRTL 5 and pituitary GM3 cells. J Endocrinol 127: 39–46

Bond J, Dawson T, Lemoine N, Wynford-Thomas D (1992) Effect of serum growth factors and phorbol ester on growth and survival of human thyroid epithelial cells expressing mutant ras. Mol Carcinog 5: 129–135

Bourke JR, Murdoch S, Manley SW, Matainaho T, Huxham GJ, Waters MJ (1991) Epidermal growth factor (EGF) inhibits the secretomotor response of the thyroid: effects of EGF on radioiodine turnover and fluid transport in cultured porcine thyroid cells. J Endocrinol 128: 213–218

Brandi ML, Rotella CM, Mavilia C, Franceschelli F, Tanini A, Toccafondi R (1987) Insulin stimulates cell growth of a new strain of differentiated rat thyroid cells. Mol Cell Endocrinol 54: 91–103

Brenner-Gati L, Berg KA, Gershengorn MC (1989) Insulin-like growth factor-I potentiates thyrotropin stimulation of adenylyl cyclase in FRTL-5 cells. Endocrinology 125: 1315–1320

Browne CA (1991) Epidermal growth factor and transforming growth factor α. In: Robertson DM, Herington AC (eds) Clinical endocrinology and metabolism, vol 5/4. Baillière Tindall, London, pp 727–754

Chanoine JP, Stein GS, Braverman LE, Shalhoub V, Lian JB, Huber CA, De Vito WJ (1992) Acidic fibroblast growth factor modulates gene expression in the rat thyroid in vivo. J Cell Biochem 50: 392–399

Cheifetz S, Hernandez H, Laiho M, ten Dijke P, Iwata KK, Massague J (1990) Distinct transforming growth factor-beta (TGF-beta) receptor subsets as determinants of cellular responsiveness to three TGF-beta isoforms. J Biol Chem 265: 20533–20538

Cirafici AM, Pepe S, Mincione G, Esposito D, Colletta G (1992) TGF beta inhibits rat thyroid cell proliferation without alterations in the expression of TSH-induced cell cycle-related genes. Biochem Biophys Res Commun 187: 225–233

Coclet J, Fourneau F, Ketelbant P, Galand P, Dumont JE (1989) Cell population kinetics in dog and human adult thyroid. Clin Endocrinol (Oxf) 31: 655–665

Cohen S (1962) Isolation of a mouse submaxillary gland protein accelerating incisor eruption and eyelid opening in the new-born animal. J Biol Chem 237: 1555–11562

Colin I, Berbinschi A, Denef JF, Ketelslegers JM (1992) Detection and identification of endothelin-1 immunoreactivity in rat and porcine thyroid follicular cells. Endocrinology 130: 544–546

Colletta G, Cirafici AM, Di Carlo A (1989) Dual effect of transforming growth factor beta on rat thyroid cells: inhibition of thyrotropin-induced proliferation and reduction of thyroid-specific differentiation markers. Cancer Res 49: 3457–3462

Colletta G, Cirafici AM, Di Carlo A, Ciardiello F, Salomon DS, Vecchio G (1991) Constitutive expression of transforming growth factor alpha does not transform rat thyroid epithelial cells. Oncogene 6: 583–587

Cowin AJ, Bidey SP (1992) Transforming growth factor-beta 1 synthesis in human thyroid follicular cells: differential effects of iodide and plasminogen on the production of latent and active peptide forms. J Endocrinol 141: 183–190

Cowin AJ, Davis JR, Bidey SP (1992) Transforming growth factor-beta 1 production in porcine thyroid follicular cells: regulation by intrathyroidal organic iodine. J Mol Endocrinol 9: 301–308

Czech MP (1989) Signal transmission by the insulin-like growth factor. Cell 59: 235–238

Dawson TP, Wyllie FS, Wynford-Thomas D (1991) In vitro responsiveness to serum growth factors is inversely related to in vivo malignancy in human thyroid epithelial cells. Br J Cancer 63: 897–900

De Larco JE, Todaro GJ (1978) Growth factors from murine sarcoma virus-transformed cells. Proc Natl Acad Sci USA 74: 4001–4005

De Vito WJ, Chanoine JP, Alex S, Fang SL, Stone S, Huber CA, Shalhoub V, Lian JB, Stein GS, Braverman LE (1992) Effect of in vivo administration of recombinant acidic fibroblast growth factor on thyroid function in the rat: induction of colloid goiter. Endocrinology 131: 729–735

Derynck R (1990) Transforming growth factor-alpha. Mol Reprod Dev 27: 3–9

Di Carlo A, Mariano A, Pisrano A, Parmeggiani U, Beguinot L, Macchia V (1990) Epidermal growth factor receptor and thyrotropin response in human thyroid tissues. J Endocrinol Invest 13: 293–299

Diamant M, Kayser L, Rasmussen AK, Bech K, Feldt-Rasmussen U (1991) Interleukin-1 is stimulated by TSH in human thyroid cells. Autoimmunity 11: 21–26

Dremier S, Taton M, Coulonval K, Nakamura T, Matsumoto K, Dumont JE (1994) Mitogenic, dedifferentiating, and scattering effects of hepatocyte growth factor on dog thyroid cells. Endocrinology 135: 135–140

Dumont JE, Maenhaut C, Pirson I, Baptist M, Roger PP (1991) Growth factors controlling the thyroid gland. In: Robertson DM, Herington AC (eds) Clinical endocrinology and metabolism, vol 5/4. Baillière Tindall, London, pp 727–754

Eggo MC,Bachrach JL, Fayet G, Burrow GN (1984) The effects of growth factors and serum on DNA synthesis and differentiation in thyroid cells in culture. Mol Cell Endocrinol 38: 141–150

Eggo MC, Sheppard MC (1994) Autocrine growth factors produced in the thyroid. Mol Cell Endocrinol 100: 97–102

Eggo MC, Pratt C, Becks GP, Burrow GN (1989) Regulation of growth and differentiation in follicle cells. Adv Exp Med Biol 261: 341–356

Eggo MC, Bachrach LK, Burrow GN (1990) Interaction of TSH, insulin and insulin-like growth factors in regulating thyroid growth and function. Growth Factors 2: 99–109

Emoto N, Isozaki O, Arai M, Murakami H, Shizume K, Baird A, Tsushima T, Demura H (1991) Identification and characterization of basic fibroblast growth factor in porcine thyroids. Endocrinology 128: 58–64

Euguchi K, Kawakami A, Nakashima M, Ida H, Sakito S, Sakai M, Terada K, Kawabe Y, Fukuda T, Ishikawa N (1993) Stimulation of mitogenesis in human thyroid epithelial cells by endothelin. Acta Endocrinol (Copenh) 128: 215–220

Fisher DA, Lakshmanan J (1990) Metabolism and effects of epidermal growth factor and related growth factors in mammals. Endocr Rev 11: 418–442

Flaumenhaft R, Abe M, Mignatti P, Rifkin DB (1992) Basic fibroblast growth factor-induced activation of latent transforming growth factor beta in endothelial cells: regulation of plasminogen activator activity. J Cell Biol 118: 901–909

Frauman AG, Moses AC (1990) Oncogenes and growth factors in thyroid carcinogenesis. Endocrinol Metab Clin North Am 19: 479–493

Gärtner R (1992) Thyroid growth in vitro. Exp Clin Endocrinol 100: 32–35

Gärtner R, Bechtner G (1990) Advances in pathogenesis of goitre. Thyroidol Clin Exp 2: 93–98

Gärtner T, Greil W, Demhardter P, Horn K (1985) Involvement of cyclic AMP, iodine and metabolites of arachidonic acid in the regulation of cell proliferation of isolated porcine thyroid follicles. Mol Cell Endocrinol 42: 145–155

Gärtner R, Bechtner G, Stübner D, Greil W (1987) Paracrine interaction between thyrocytes and fibroblasts. Acta Endocrinol (Copenh) 281: 225–230

Gärtner R, Bechtner G, Stübner D, Greil W (1990) Growth regulation of porcine thyroid follicles in vitro by growth factors. Horm Metab Res Suppl 23: 61–67

Goretzki PE, Koob R, Koller T, Simon R, Branscheid D, Clark OH (1986) The effect of thyrotropin and cAMP on DNA synthesis and cell growth of human thyrocytes in monolayer culture. Surgery 100: 1053–1061

Gorgoulis V, Aninos D, Priftis C, Evagelopoulou C, Karameris A, Kanavaros P, Spandidos DA (1992) Expression of epidermal growth factor, transforming growth factor-alpha and epidermal growth factor receptor in thyroid tumors. In Vivo 6: 291–296

Gospodarowicz D, Neufield G, Schweigerer L (1986) Fibroblast growth factors. Mol Cell Endocrinol 46: 187–204

Gregory H (1975) Isolation and structure of urogastrone and its relationship to epidermal growth factor. Nature 275: 325–327

Greil W, Rafferzeder M, Bechtner G, Gärtner R (1989) Release of an endothelial cell growth factor from cultured porcine thyroid follicles. Mol Endocrinol 3: 858–865

Grubeck-Loebenstein B, Buchan G, Sadeghi R, Kissonerghis M, Londei M, Turner M, Pirich K, Roka R, Niederle B, Kassal H et al (1989) Transforming growth factor beta regulates thyroid growth. Role in the pathogenesis of nontoxic goiter. J Clin Invest 83: 764–770

Haugen DR, Aksen LA, Varhaug JE, Lillehaug JR (1993) Demonstration of a TGF-alpha-EGF-receptor autocrine loop and c-myc protien overexpression in papillary thyroid carcinomas. Int J Cancer 55: 37–43

Hearn MTW (1991) Structure and function of heparin-binding (fibroblast) growth factor family. In: Robertson DM, Herington AC (eds) Clinical endocrinology and metabolism, vol 5/4. Baillière Tindall, London, pp 571–593
Heldin NE, Westermark B (1988) Epidermal growth factor, but not thyrotropin, stimulates the expression of c-fos and c-myc messenger ribonucleic acid in porcine thyroid follicle cells in primary culture. Endocrinology 122: 1042–1046
Heldin NE, Cvejic D, Smeds S, Westermark B (1991) Coexpression of functionally active receptors for thyrotropin and platelet-derived growth factor in human thyroid carcinoma cells. Endocrinology 129: 2187–2193
Herington AC (1991) Insulin-like growth factors: biochemistry and physiology. In: Robertson DM, Herington AC (eds) Clinical endocrinology and metabolism, vol 5/4. Baillière Tindall, London, pp 727–754
Hoermann R, Saller B, Mann K (1989) Insulin and insulin-like growth factor (IGF I) modulate the effects of bTSH on 3H-thymidine incorporation in human thyroid cells in primary culture. Klin Wochenschr 67: 976–979
Hofbauer LC, Rafferzeder M, Janssen OE (1995) Insulin-like growth factor-1 messenger ribonucleic acid expression in porcine thyroid follicles is regulated by thyrotropin, epidermal growth factor and iodine. Eur J Endocrinol 132: 605–610
Hsuan JJ, Panayotou G, Waterfield MD (1989) Structural basis for epidermal growth factor receptor function. Prog Growth Factor Res 1: 23–32
Jackson S, Tseng YC, Lahiri S, Burman KD, Wartofsky L (1992) Receptors for endothelin in cultured human thyroid cells and inhibition by endothelin of thyroglobulin secretion. J Clin Endocrinol Metab 75: 388–392
Kanamori A, Abe Y, Yajima Y, Manabe Y, Ito K (1989) Epidermal growth factor receptors in plasma membranes of normal and diseased human thyroid glands. J Clin Endocrinol Metab 68: 899–903
Kodama M, Daa T, Kashima K, Yokoyama S, Nakayama I, Noguchi S (1994) Immunohistochemical localization of acid and basic fibroblast growth factor in human benign and malignant thyroid lesions. Jpn J Clin Oncol 24: 66–73
Kraiem Z, Sadeh O, Sobel E (1990) Thyrotropin acting at least partially via adenosine 3′,5′monophosphate, exerts both mitogenic and antimitogenic effects in cultured human thyroid cells. J Clin Endocrinol Metab 70: 497–502
Lemoine NR, Hughes CM, Gullick WJ, Brown CL, Wynford-Thomas D (1991) Abnormalities of the EGF receptor system in human thyroid neoplasia. Int J Cancer 49: 558–561
Lewinski A (1981) Pituitary is not required for compensatory hyperplasia. Horm Res 15: 287–412
Lewinski A, Bartke A, Smith NKR (1993a) Compensatory thyroid hyperplasia in hemithyroidectomized snell dwarf mice. Endocrinology 113: 3217–2319
Lewinski A, Pawlikowski M, Cardinali DP (1993b) Thyroid growth stimulating and growth inhibiting factors. Biol Signals 2: 313–351
Logan A, Black EG, Gonzalez AM, Buscaglia M, Sheppard MC (1992) Basic fibroblast growth factor: an autocrine mitogen of rat thyroid follicular cells? Endocrinology 130: 2363–2372
Logan A, Smith C, Becks GP, Gonzalez AM, Phillips ID, Hill DJ (1994) Enhanced expression of transforming growth factor-beta 1 during thyroid hyperplasia in rats. J Endocrinol 141: 45–57
Maciel RMB, Moses AC, Villone G, Tramontano D, Ingbar SH (1988) Demonstration of the production and physiological role of insulin-like growth factor II in rat thyroid follicular cells in culture. J Clin Invest 82: 1546–1553
Mak WW, Eggo MC, Burrow GN (1984) Thyrotropin regulation of plasminogen activity in primary cultures of ovine thyroid cells. Biochem Biophys Res Commun 123: 633–640
Makinen T, Pekonen F, Franssila K, Lanmberg BA (1988) Receptors for epidermal growth factor and thyrotropin in thyroid carcinoma. Acta Endocrinol (Copenh) 117: 45–50
Many MC, Denef JF, Haumont S (1984) Precocity of the endothelial proliferation during a course of rapid goitrogenesis. Acta Endocrinol (Copenh) 105: 487–491
Minuto F, Barreca A, Del Monte P, Cariola G, Torre GC, Giordano G (1989) Immunoreactive insulin-like growth factor I (IGF-I) and IGF-I-binding protein content in human thyroid tissue. J Clin Endocrinol Metab 68: 621–626

Miyamoto M, Sugawa H, Kuma K, Mori T, Imura H (1989) Analysis of epidermal growth factor (EGF) receptor and effect of EGF on the growth of cultured Graves' and non-neoplastic human thyroid cells. J Endocrinol Invest 12: 111–117

Mizukami Y, Nonomura A, Hashimoto T, Michigishi T, Noguchi M, Matsubara F, Yanaihara N (1991) Immunohistochemical demonstration of epidermal growth factor and c-myc oncogene product in normal, benign and malignant thyroid tissues. Histopathology 18: 11–18

Moris JC III, Ranganathan G, Hay ID, Nelson RE, Jiang NS (1988) The effects of transforming growth factor-β on growth and differentiation of the continuous rat follicular cell line, FRTL-5. Endocrinology 123: 1385–1394

Nolte A, Bechtner G, Rafferzeder M, Gärtner R (1994) Interleukin-1 beta binds to intact porcine thyroid follicles, decreases iodide uptake but has no effect on cAMP formation or proliferation. Horm Metab Res 26: 413–418

Ooi GT, Herington AC (1988) The biological and structural characterization of specific serum binding proteins for insulin-like growth factors. J Endocrinol 118: 7–18

Ollis CA, Hill DJ, Munro DS (1989) A role for insulin-like growth factor-I in the regulation of human thyroid cell growth by thyrotropin. J Clin Endocrinol Metab 123: 95–500

Onoda N, Ohmura E, Tsushima T, Ohba Y, Emoto N, Isozaki O, Sato Y, Shizume K, Demura H (1992) Autocrine role of insulin-like growth factor (IGF)-I in a human thyroid cancer cell line. Eur J Cancer 28A: 1904–1909

Ozawa S, Spaulding SW (1990) Epidermal growth factor inhibits radioiodine uptake but stimulates deoxyribonucleic acid synthesis in newborn rat thyroids grown in nude mice. Endocrinology 127: 604–612

Pang XP, Hershman JM (1990) Differential effects of growth factors on [^{3}H]thymidine incorporation and [^{125}I]iodine uptake in FRTL-5 rat thyroid cells. Proc Soc Exp Biol Med 194: 240–244

Pang XP, Park M, Hershman JM (1992) Transforming growth factor-beta blocks protein kinase-A-mediated iodide transport and protein kinase-C-mediated DNA synthesis in FRTL-5 rat thyroid cells. Endocrinology 131: 45–50

Parma J, Duprez L, Van Sande J, Cochaux P, Gervy C, Mockel J, Dumont J, Vassart G (1993) Somatic mutations in the thyrotropin receptor gene cause hyperfunctioning thyroid adenomas. Nature 365: 49–51

Phillips ID, Becks GP, Wang JF, Han VK, Hill DJ (1994) Hormonal regulation and biological actions of insulin-like growth factor binding proteins in isolated ovine thyroid follicles. Endocrinology 134: 1238–1246

Pratt MAC, Eggo MC, Bachrach LK, Craayon P, Burrow GN (1989) Regulation of thyroperoxidase, thyroglobulin and iodide levels in sheep thyroid cells by TSH, tumor promoters and epidermal growth factor. Biochimie 71: 227–235

Purchino A, Cooper J, Brunner A, Lioubin M, Gentry L, Kovacina K, Roth R, Marquardt H (1988) Identification of mannose-6-phosphate in two asparagine-linked sugar chains of recombinant transforming growth factor-β_1 precursor. J Biol Chem 263: 14211–14215

Rafferzeder M, Hofbauer L, Janssen O, Bechtner G, Gärtner R (1993) Thyrotropin stimulated IGF-I mRNA expression in isolated porcine thyroid follicles is under negative control of iodine. J Endocrinol Invest 16 Suppl 2: 110

Raspe E, Reuse S, Maenhaut C, Roger PP, Corvilain B, Laurent E, Mockel F, Lamy F, Van Sande J, Dumont JE (1989) Importance and variability of transducing systems in the control of thyroid cell function, proliferation and differentiation. Front Horm Res 18: 1–13

Roberts AB, Sporn MB (1990) The transforming growth factor-β. In: Sporn MB, Roberts AB (eds) Peptide growth factors and their receptors, vol 2. Springer, Berlin Heidelberg New York, pp 419–472

Robertson DM (1991) Transforming growth factor β/inhibin family. In: Robertson DM, Herington AC (eds) Clinical endocrinology and metabolism, vol 5/4. Baillière Tindall, London, pp 727–754

Roger PP, Dumont JE (1982) Epidermal growth factor controls the proliferation and the expression of differentiation in canine thyroid cells in primary culture. FEBS Lett 144: 209–212

Roger PP, Dumont JE (1984) Factors controlling proliferation and differentiation of canine thyroid cells cultured in reduced serum conditions: effects of thyrotropin, cyclic AMP and growth factors. Mol Cell Endocrinol 36: 79–93

Rognoni JB, Penel C, Gostein J, Galand P, Dumont JE (1987) Cell kinetics of thyroid epithelial cells during hyperplastic goitre involution. J Endocrinol 114: 483–490

Santisteban P, Acebron A, Polycarpou-Schwarz M, Di Lauro R (1992) Insulin and insulin-like growth factor I regulate a thyroid-specific nuclear protein that binds to the thyroglobulin promoter. Mol Endocrinol 6: 1310–1317

Smith P, Wynford-Thomas D, Stringer BMJ, Williams ED (1986) Growth factor control of rat thyroid follicular cell proliferation. Endocrinology 119: 1439–1445

Song B (1991) Immunohistochemical demonstration of epidermal growth factor receptor and ceruloplasmin in thyroid diseases. Acta Pathol Jpn 41: 336–343

Stübner D, Gärtner R, Greil W, Gropper K, Brabant G, Permanetter W, Horn K, Pickardt CR (1987) Hypertrophy and hyperplasia during goitre growth and involution in rats – separate bioeffect of TSH and iodine. Acta Endocrinol (Copenh) 116: 537–548

Sugenoya A, Masuda H, Komatsu M, Yokoyama S, Shimizu T, Fujimori M, Kobayashi S, Iida F (1992) Adenomatous goitre: therapeutic strategy, postoperative outcome, and study of epidermal growth factor receptor. Br J Surg 79: 404–406

Takasu N, Takasu M, Komiya I, Nagasawa Y, Asawa T, Shimizu Y, Yamada T (1989) Insulin-like growth factor I stimulates inositol phosphate accumulation, a rise in cytoplasmic free calcium, and proliferation in cultured porcine thyroid cells. J Biol Chem 264: 18485–18488

Taton M, Lamy F, Roger PP, Dumont JE (1993) General inhibition by transforming growth factor beta 1 of thyrotropin and cAMP responses in human thyroid cells in primary culture. Mol Cell Endocrinol 95: 13–21

Taylor AH, Millatt LJ, Whitley GS, Johnstone AP, Nussey SS (1993) The effect of basic fibroblast growth factor on the growth and function of human thyrocytes. J Endocrinol 136: 339–344

Thomas KA, Gimenez-Gallego G (1986) Fibroblast growth factors: broad spectrum mitogens with potent angiogenic activity. Trends Biochem Sci 11: 81–84

Todd I, Hammond LJ, James RF, Feldmann M, Bottazzo GF (1990) Epidermal growth factor and transforming growth factor-alpha suppress HLA class II induction in human thyroid epithelial cells. Immunology 69: 91–96

Tode B, Serio M, Rotella CM, Galli G, Franceschelli F, Tanini A, Toccafondi R (1989) Insulin-like growth factor-I: autocrine secretion by human thyroid follicular cells in primary culture. J Clin Endocrinol Metab 69: 639–647

Tohyama K, Yoshida Y, Ohashi K, Sano E, Kobayashi H, Endo K, Naruto M, Nakamura T (1992) Production of multiple growth factors by a newly established human thyroid carcinoma cell line. Jpn J Cancer Res 83: 153–158

Tramontano D, Cushing G, Moses AC, Ingbar SH (1986) Insulin-like growth factor-I stimulates the growth of rat thyroid cells in culture and synergizes the stimulation of DNA synthesis induced by TSH and Graves' IgG. Endocrinology 119: 940–942

Tseng YC, Burman KD, Schaudies RP, Ahmann AJ, D'Avis J, Geelhoed GW, Wartofsky L (1989) Effects of epidermal growth factor on thyroglobulin and adenosine 3′,5′-monophosphate production by cultured human thyrocytes. J Clin Endocrinol Metab 69: 771–775

Tseng YC, Lahiri S, Jackson S, Burman KD, Wartofsky L (1993) Endothelin binding to receptors and endothelin production by human thyroid follicular cells: effect of transforming growth factor-beta and thyrotropin. J Clin Endocrinol Metab 76: 156–161

Tsushima T, Arai M, Saji M et al (1988) Effects of transforming growth factor-β on deoxyribonucleic acid synthesis and iodine metabolism in porcine thyroid cells in culture. Endocrinology 123: 1187–1194

Usuki K, Heldin NE, Miyazono K, Ishikawa F, Takaku F, Westermark B, Heldin CH (1989) Production of platelet-derived endothelial cell growth factor by normal and transformed human cells in culture. Proc Natl Acad Sci USA 86: 7427–7431

Vannelli GB, Barni T, Modigliani U, Paulin I, Serio M, Maggi M, Fiorelli G, Balboni GC (1990) Insulin-like growth factor-I receptors in nonfunctioning thyroid nodules. J Clin Endocrinol Metab 71: 1175–1182

Veneziani BM, Di Marino C, Salvatore P, Villone G, Perrotti N, Frunzio R, Tramontano D (1992) Transfected insulin-like growth factor II modulates the mitogenic response of rat thyrocytes in culture. Mol Cell Endocrinol 86: 11–20

Wang JF, Becks GP, Buckingham KD, Hill DJ (1990) Characterization of insulin-like growth factor-binding proteins secreted by isolated sheep thyroid epithelial cells. J Endocrinol 125: 439–448

Watanabe Y, Amino N, Tamaki H, Iwatani Y, Miyai K (1985) Bovine thyrotropin inhibits DNA synthesis inversely with stimulation of cyclic AMP production in cultured porcine thyroid cells. Endocrinol Jpn 32: 81–88

Waters MJ, Tweedale RC, Whip TA et al (1987) Dedifferentiation of cultured thyroid cells by epidermal growth factor: some insights into the mechanism. Mol Cell Endocrinol 49: 109–117

Westermark B, Karlsson FA, Walinder O (1978) Thyrotropin is not a growth factor for human thyroid cells in culture. Proc Natl Acad Sci USA 76: 2022–2026

Westermark K, Karlsson FA, Westermark B (1983) Epidermal growth factor modulates thyroid growth and function in culture. Endocrinology 112: 1680–1686

Westermark K, Westermark B, Karlsson FA, Ericson LE (1986) Localisation of epidermal growth factor receptors on porcine thyroid follicle cells and receptor regulation by thyrotropin. Endocrinology 118: 1040–1046

Williams DW, Wynford-Thomas D, Williams ED (1987) Control of human thyroid follicular cell proliferation in suspension and monolayer culture. Mol Cell Endocrinol 51: 33–40

Williams DW, Williams ED, Wynford-Thomas D (1989) Evidence for autocrine production of IGF-1 in human thyroid adenomas. Mol Cell Endocrinol 61: 139–145

Wuester C, Steger G, Schmelze A, Gottswinter J, Minne HW, Ziegler R (1991) Increased incidence of euthyroid and hyperthyroid goiter independently of thyrotropin in patients with acromegaly. Horm Metab Res 23: 131–134

Wyllie FS, Dawson T, Bond JA, Goretzki P, Game S, Prime S, Wynford-Thomas D (1991) Correlated abnormalities of transforming growth factor-beta 1 response and p53 expression in thyroid epithelial cell transformation. Mol Cell Endocrinol 76: 13–21

Wynford-Thomas D, Smith P, Williams ED (1987) Proliferative response to cyclic AMP elevation of thyroid epithelium in suspension culture. Mol Cell Endocrinol 51: 163–166

Yashiro T, Tsushima T, Murakami H, Obara T, Fujimoto Y, Shizume K, Ito K (1991) Insulin-like growth factor-II (IGF-II)/mannose-6-phosphate receptors are increased in primary human thyroid neoplasms. Eur J Cancer 27:699–703

Yashiro T, Arai M, Shizume K, Obara T, Murakami H, Hizuka N, Emoto N, Miyakawa M, Ito K, Tsushima T (1994) Increased activity of insulin-like growth factor-binding protein in human thyroid papillary cancer tissue. Jpn J Cancer Res 85: 46–62

Yasui W, Ji ZQ, Kuniyasu H, Ayhan A, Yokozaki H, Ito H, Tahara E (1992) Expression of transforming growth factor alpha in human tissues: immunohistochemical study and northern blot analysis. Virchows Arch [A] 421: 513–519

Yuasa R, Eggo MC, Meinkoth J, Dillmann WH, Burrow GN (1992) Iodide induces transforming growth factor beta 1 (TGF-beta 1) mRNA in sheep thyroid cells. Thyroid 2: 141–145

Zerek-Melen G, Lewinski A, Szkudlinski M (1990) Influence of somatostatin and epidermal growth factor (EGF) on the proliferation of thyroid follicular cells in organ culture. Regul Pept 28: 293–300

Thyroid Carcinoma: Interrelationships Between Local Thyroid Hormone Metabolism by the Type I 5′-Deiodinase and the Expression of Thyroid Hormone Receptors and Other Thyroid-Specific (De-)differentiation Markers

J. Köhrle

1 Local Thyroid Hormone Production and Action in the Thyroid

1.1 Thyroid Hormone Deiodination

The human thyroid and the thyroid glands of most other species which produce thyroid hormones express high levels of type I 5′-deiodinase (5′-DI), the isoenzyme that catalyses the deiodination of the prohormone L-thyroxine (3,3′5,5′-tetraiodo-L-thyronine, T_4) to the biologically active form 3,3′,5-triiodo-L-thyronine (L-T_3) (Fig. 1). Expression of the second isozyme, type II 5′-deiodinase (5′-DII), which catalyses the same reaction but with different biochemical charac-

Current Topics in Pathology
Volume 91, K.W. Schmid/W. Böcker (Eds.)

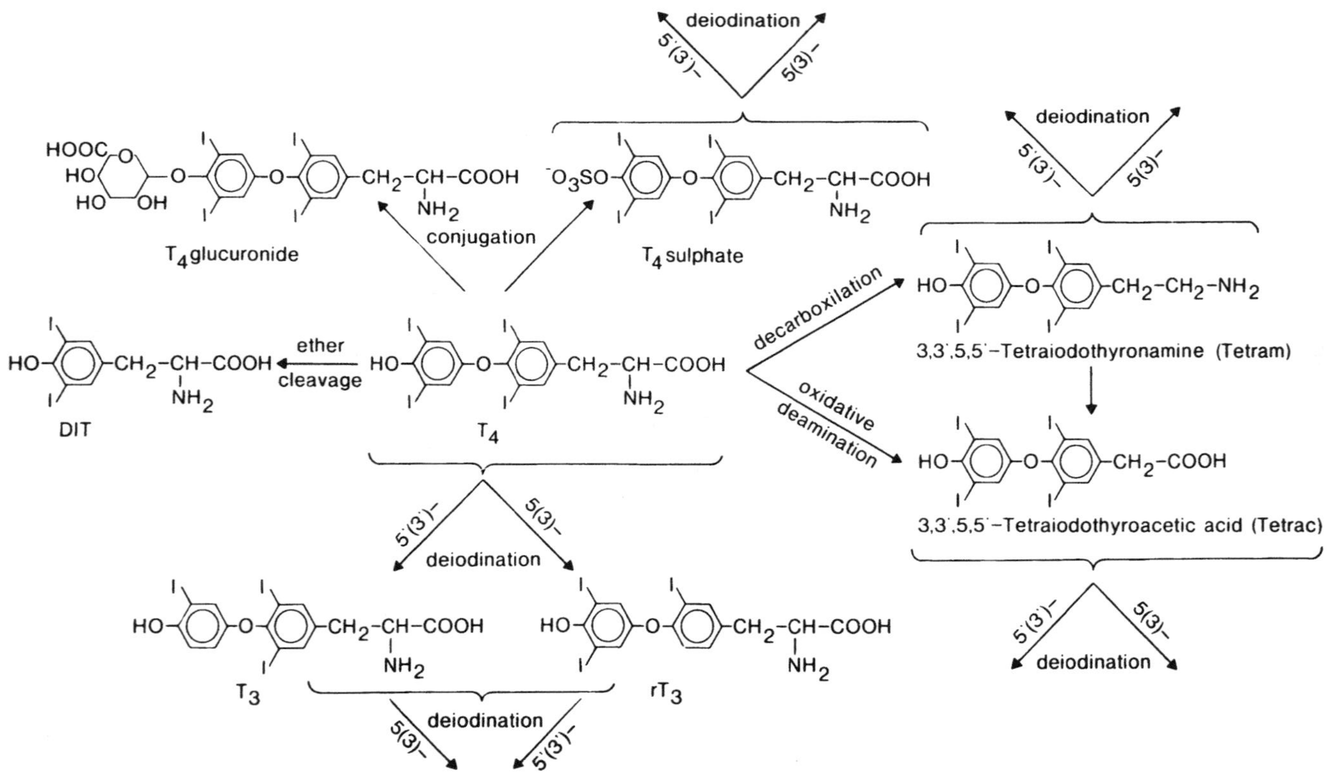

Fig. 1. Pathways of thyroid hormone (T_4) metabolism

teristics, has been ruled out in thyroid tissues (for review see (KÖHRLE 1994a)). So far, no evidence for the presence of the third deiodinase isozyme, 5-deiodinase (5-D), in thyroid tissue has been presented either. 5-D catalyses the inactivation of T_4, T_3, and other iodothyronines by removing iodine atoms from the 5- or 3-position of the tyrosyl ring of iodothyronines. Under certain in vitro reaction conditions, such as alkaline pH, 5′-DI is also able to remove iodine atoms from the tyrosyl ring, due to a certain "wobble" in the active site, possibly induced by a pH-dependent alteration of the imidazolium selenolate ion pair in the active site of 5′-DI (KÖHRLE et al. 1991; KÖHRLE 1994a). However, in vivo, 5′-DI is rather specific for the removal of iodine atoms from the 5′- (or chemically equivalent 3′-) position of the phenolic ring. 5′-DI is solely found in the thyrocytes, not in calcitonin-producing C cells (BOYE and LAURBERG 1984). Like the other tissues and isozymes, thyroid 5′-DI is also an integral membrane protein, but its subcellular location in the thyrocyte has not yet been studied. Several human and rat thyroid cell lines in culture express 5′-DI (Table 1) which allows the mechanism of thyroid-specific expression and regulation of 5′-DI activity to be studied (SCHRECK et al. 1994; KÖHRLE 1994a).

1.2 Regulation of 5′-DI Expression in the Thyrocyte

1.2.1 Thyroid-Stimulating Hormone

The regulation of 5′-DI in the human thyroid is different to that in liver, kidney, the euthyroid pituitary and euthyroid brain (Table 2) (KÖHRLE 1990, 1994a; ISHII et al. 1981, 1982, 1983; SUGAWARA et al. 1984). 5′-DI expression and activity is induced in all of these tissues, including the thyroid, under hyperthyroid conditions. During hypothyroidism, however, 5′-DI activity is reduced in liver, kidney, pituitary and brain, whereas in thyroid tissue 5′-DI expression is induced. Several groups have shown in various animal models, tissue slices, perfused thyroid tissue and cell culture that expression of thyroid 5′-DI is under the positive control of TSH (ISHII et al. 1983; ERICKSON et al. 1982; WU 1983; KUBOTA et al. 1984; WU et al. 1985; LAURBERG 1981; PEETERS et al. 1992) which is elevated under conditions of hypothyroidism and severe iodine deficiency (GREER et al. 1968; MASHITA et al. 1982; KÖHRLE 1990). 5′-DI expression is stimulated via the TSH-receptor-Gsα-protein-adenylate cyclase-cAMP signal transduction pathway and the induction can be blocked by transcription and translation inhibitors (ISHII et al. 1983; KÖHRLE 1990, 1994a). It must be postulated that the thyroid-specific 5′-DI promotor contains a cAMP-responsive element (CRE) or is activated by another cAMP-dependent process. Therefore, it must be assumed that under hypothyroid conditions, where TSH is elevated, the thyroid production of T_3 from T_4 is increased in a similar way to the augmented T_3 production during hyperthyroidism. Stimulation of 5′-DI activity was also demonstrated by administration of stimulating Graves' immunoglobulins, which also act via the TSH-receptor pathway (ISHII et al. 1981; WU et al. 1987; TOYODA et al. 1990). T_3 secretion after stimulation of porcine thyroid slices is a much more sensitive parameter for thyroid-stimulating

Table 1. Currently established and characterized human and animal thyroid cell lines

Cell line	Established	Origin, tumour type	TSH receptor	TSH response	Tg	TPO	5′-DI	Growth factor/receptor	Chromosomal abnormalities	Reference
FTC-133[a]	Cell culture	♂, lymph node metastasis follicular carcinoma	+	+	+		+	EGF-R	+	GORETZKI et al. (1990)
FTC-236[a]	Cell culture	♂, neck lymph node metastasis follicular carcinoma					(+)		+	GORETZKI et al. (1990)
FTC-238[a]	Cell culture	♂, lung metastasis follicular carcinoma					(+)		+	GORETZKI et al. (1990)
C643	Cell culture	76 y ♂, anaplastic carcinoma	–	–	+	–	–	PDGF-R	+	HELDIN (1988)
HTh 74	3 passages onto athymic mice	73 y ♀, anaplastic carcinoma	+	+	(+)	–	–	PDGF-R		HELDIN (1991)
HTC/C3	Cell culture	44 y ♀, undifferentiated carcinoma	–	–	+	+	–	EGF-R, secretes growth factors		ENOMOTO (1990)
SGHTL-34	SV3neo transformed	Normal human thyroid cells	+	+						WHITLEY (1987)
NIM 1	Cell culture	Metastatic papillary carcinoma	–	–	+			IL-1-R, secretes IL-1α and β		KOBAYASHI (1989)
RO 87-M-1		Follicular carcinoma						SSt-R		ESTOUR (1989)

RO 82-W-1		Follicular carcinoma	–	–				SSt-R	Estour (1989)
RO 90-D-1		Anaplastic carcinoma						SSt-R	Estour (1989)
NPA 87		Papillary carcinoma						SSt-R	Estour (1989)
KAK-1		Follicular adenoma						SSt-R	Ain et al. (1992)
KAT-4		Anaplastic carcinoma						SSt-R	Ain et al. (1992)
WRO	hTSH-R transfection of RO 82-W-1		+	–					Namba et al. (1993)
HTC	hTSH-R transfection of FTC-133		+	+					Derwahl et al. (1933)
FRTL-5	Cell culture	Rat thyroid	+	+	+	+	+		Ambesi-Impiombato (1980)
PORTHOS	Cell cuture	Porcine							Hovsépiant (1993)
ATHOS	Cell culture derived from PORTHOS	Porcine	+	+					Hovsépian (1993)
OVNIS-5H	Cell culture	Sheep							Hovsépian (1986)
PETCAT	Cell culture	Cat							Gerber (1989)

[a] Established from sequential metastases of a follicular thyroid carcinoma in the same patient.
TSH, Thyroid-stimulating hormone; Tg, thyroglobulin; TPO, thyroperoxidase; EGF, epidermal growth factor; PDGF, platelet-derived growth factor; SSt, somatostatin; R, receptor; +, expressed; –, not expressed.

Table 2. Tissue-specific expression and regulation of deiodinase isozymes

Property	Type I 5′-deiodinase	Type II 5′-deiodinase	5-Deiodinase
Substrate preference	$rT_3 >> T_4 >> T_3$	$T_4 > rT_3 >> T_3$	$T_3 \geq T_4$; sulfates > phenolates
Reaction kinetics	Ping-pong	Sequential	Sequential
Active site residues	Selenocysteine, histidine	Cysteine	Cysteine?
Subunits (kDa)	27 000, selenoprotein	29 000	?
Holoenzyme	52 000	200 000	?
Tissue distribution	Thyroid, liver, kidney, euthyroid CNS	(Hypothyroid) CNS, anterior pituitary, brown adipose tissue, placenta	CNS, most tissues except anterior pituitary
Subcellular location	Liver: endoplasmic reticulum kidney: basal-lateral plasma membrane	Microsomal membranes	Microsomal membranes
Inhibitors: Thiouracils	+ + +	(+)	(+)
Iopanoate	+ + +	+ + +	+ + +
Iodoacetate	+ + +	+	?
Hyperthyroidism	Increased activity	Decreased activity	Increased activity
Hypothyroidism	Decreased activity	Increased activity	Decreased activity
Low-T3 syndrome	Decreased activity	No change	?

+ + +, Strong inhibition; (+) very weak inhibition.

Graves' immunoglobulins than T_4 secretion (ATKINSON and KENDALL-TAYLOR 1981; HÖRMANN et al. 1990). In primary cultures of human thyroid cells in the presence of 10% fetal calf serum, TSH and TSAb acutely stimulate cAMP production and secretion into the medium via the TSH-receptor pathway (KRAIEM et al. 1991). However, a marked TSH-induced increase in T_3 secretion is only detectable 1–4 days after treatment. Propylthiouracil (PTU) blocked the TSH effect on T_3 secretion by more than 60%, but methyl-mercapto-imidazole (MMI) was also active, which is indicative of de novo synthesis of T_3 rather than secretion of preformed (T_4 or) T_3 (MASHITA et al. 1982)! In these experiments no direct indication of stimulation of human thyroid 5′-DI activity by TSH was found, but a detailed analysis of T_3/T_4 secretion ratios was not performed (KRAIEM et al. 1991). Whereas no remarkable rT_3 secretion has been reported for the human thyroid, rT_3 secretion in the dog thyroid gland, which consists of two independent lobes, amounts to 1/10 of the T_3 secreted (WESTGREN et al. 1977; LAURBERG 1980, 1981). In these studies again no evidence of TSH-dependent modification of intrathyroid iodothyronine deiodination by prolonged thyroid stimulation by TSH was found (LAURBERG 1980, 1981). However, the secretion pattern of thyroid hormones depends on intrathyroid deiodination by 5′-DI, because PTU, a potent 5′-DI inhibitor, but not MMI, an inhibitor of thyroperoxidase but not 5′-DI, markedly reduces T_3 secretion and decreases the T_3/T_4 secretion ratio (LAURBERG 1978, 1980, 1981).

Together, these in vitro studies support clinical observations of an increased secretion ratio of T_3/T_4 during both hypo- and hyperthyroidism. The elevated production of T_3 or preferential T_3 secretion so far has been attributed to an altered T_3/T_4 ratio in thyroglobulin. These recent observations on hormonally regulated alterations of the very high specific 5′-DI activity in the thyroid itself (KÖHRLE 1994a; KÖHRLE et al. 1991; SCHRECK et al. 1994; BEECH et al. 1993; CHANOINE et al. 1993) require a detailed reanalysis of the relative contribution of the local 5′-DI activity to the thyroid hormone secretion pattern, which apparently is not only determined by the altered hormone synthesis under conditions of iodine deficiency or hyperstimulation by Graves' immunoglobulins, as the textbooks say. In contrast to the effect on thyroid 5′-DI, no stimulatory effect of cAMP or glucagon (which also uses the cAMP pathway, similar to TSH) on liver 5′-DI activity was found in rat liver in several models (KÖHRLE 1994a; MÜLLER et al. 1982). Whereas alterations of intracellular pH lead to changes in liver 5′-DI activity, neither glucagon nor cAMP has an effect on 5′-DI activity and T_3 production in the isolated perfused rat liver (KÖHRLE et al. 1982; MÜLLER et al. 1982). Apparently glucagon and cAMP alter T_3 elimination in the liver. Alteration of T_3 elimination in the thyroid has not yet been observed after TSH and cAMP stimulation. Starvation affects thyroid hormone secretion and alters the T_3/T_4 ratio in circulation in the rat (WU 1990; CHANOINE et al. 1992; KINLAW et al. 1985), whereas starvation-associated alterations of the thyroid status in man do not suggest altered thyroid hormone secretion (KÖHRLE 1994a). A detailed kinetic analysis of the thyroid and peripheral contributions to T_3 production in healthy adult volunteers was published recently (PILO et al. 1990).

1.2.2 Thyroid Hormones

The mechanism of thyroid hormone-dependent stimulation of thyroid 5′-DI has not been studied in sufficient detail yet. Rat thyroid 5′-DI is stimulated by TSH (in MMI-treated rats) and reaches the limit of detection after hypophysectomy (with or without euthyroid T_4 replacement), in contrast to the 5′-DI activity of rat liver, which was reduced to one-fifth of its activity and restored to normal after euthyroid T_4 substitution of hypophysectomized rats (ERICKSON et al. 1982). This study suggested that T_4 is not able to directly induce 5′-DI in the thyroid in the absence of pituitary hormones such as GH, and that rat liver 5′-DI is under the control of thyroid hormone but not dependent on GH, whose synthesis and release is thyroid hormone-dependent in the rat. The groups of Wu and Ishii (WU 1990; WU et al. 1985; ISHII et al. 1983; KÖHRLE 1990) reached different conclusions in several studies using mouse, guinea pig and dog models. They provided evidence that thyroid 5′-DI is induced by T_4 and/or T_3 under in vivo and in vitro conditions. The latter data were supported by the cell culture studies using the differentiated rat thyroid line FRTL-5 (BORGES et al. 1990; TOYODA et al. 1992a). It remains uncertain whether species differences, pituitary hormones, GH-dependent factors such as IGF-I, which are synthesized by thyroid cells in vitro and in vivo, or serum-dependent factors contained in the culture media account for these differences. Furthermore, the use of recombinant pure species-specific TSH preparations instead of extracted, mostly bovine TSH will be necessary to exclude "adjuvant" effects of contaminants of extracted material in vivo or in cell cultures in the presence of serum. The latter statement should be considered in the context of a single report on stimulation of 5′-DI in perfused rat kidney by extracted bovine TSH preparations (IKEDA et al. 1985), as we now definitely know that kidney tissue does not express TSH receptors. The identification and functional assays of TREs (thyroid-responsive elements) and CREs in the thyroid-specific promoter of 5′-DI will solve this issue. In vivo and in vitro both T_4 and T_3, but not the inactive metabolite rT_3 or other iodothyronines without thyromimetic potency, stimulate 5′-DI activity (KÖHRLE 1994a). Some evidence suggests that stimulation occurs by enzyme induction as stated above for the TSH-cAMP effect. However, no TRE or related DNA sequence has been identified in the 5′-DI promoter, which is not yet characterized. The thyroid hormone-induced stimulation of 5′-DI activity occurs independently of the TSH-cAMP effect. However, the presence of thyroid hormone in the cell culture medium enhances the TSH-cAMP effect and vice versa, a finding to be expected for two independent mechanisms. Current opinion implies that most of the thyroid hormone effects mediated by the thyroid hormone-activated members of the nuclear receptor superfamily, the c-erbA-α (TRα) or c-erbA-β (TRβ) trans-activating factors (TAF), are mediated by T_3, but not by T_4 (KÖHRLE 1994a; CHIN et al. 1993). T_4 has to be activated to the thyromimetically active T_3 by one of the two 5′-D enzymes, type I 5′-DI in the thyroid, and cannot activate the TAFs in the nuclear compartment in vivo. It will be an experimentally difficult task to exclude a direct effect of T_4 on nuclear T_3 receptors. Therefore, the deiodinase isozymes act as "guardians of the gate" to the nuclear action of thyroid hormone and control the supply of active hormone to the nucleus (Fig. 2).

1.3 Do Deiodinase Isozymes Exert a Strategic Role for Hormone Action via Nuclear T_3 Receptors?

It will be interesting to find out where inside the cell, especially in the thyrocyte, the 5′-DI is located: in the cytosolic-oriented leaflet of the membrane of the rough and smooth endoplasmic reticulum, as in rat liver (KÖHRLE 1994a), or in the inner plasma membrane, as in kidney (LEONARD et al. 1991) and rat cerebral cortex (LEONARD et al. 1982). In all of these tissues, the active site of the enzyme is oriented toward the cytosol (KÖHRLE 1994a), but it is not yet known whether 5′-DI contributes to the transmembrane passage of the hydrophobic thyroid hormones in concert or cooperation with the plasma or nuclear membrane-associated thyroid hormone-specific transporters (RAO et al. 1981; MOORADIAN et al. 1985; BLONDEAU et al. 1988; PONTECORVI and ROBBINS 1989; KRENNING and DOCTER 1991). In the epithelial cells of the proximal kidney tubule, 5′-DI is specifically located in the basal-lateral, but not the apical inner plasma membrane (LEONARD

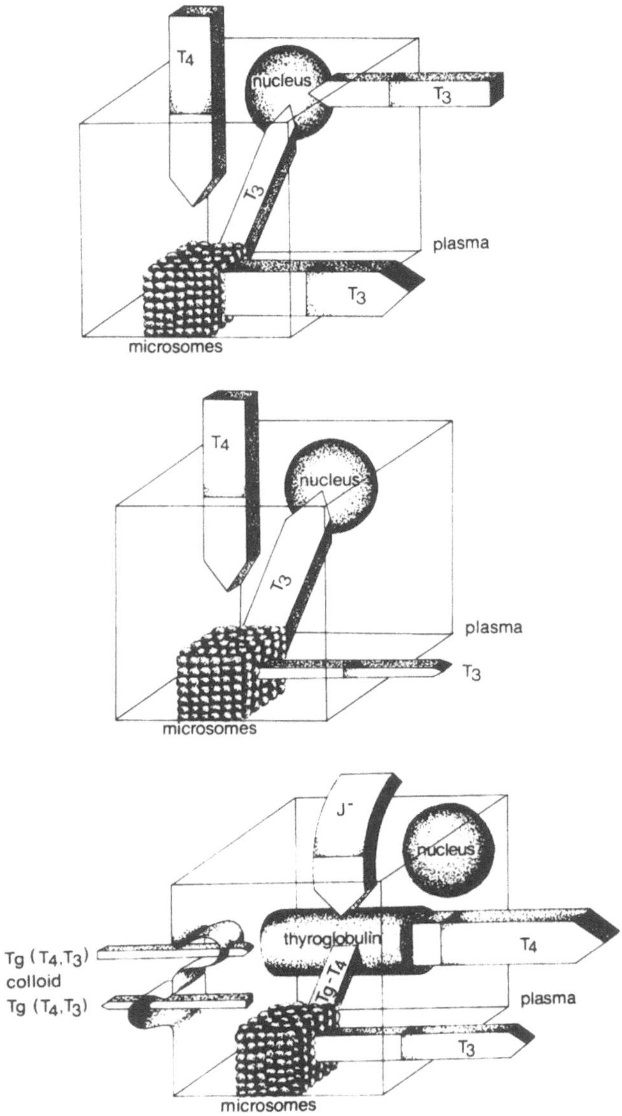

Fig. 2. The role of deiodinase enzymes in the local or systemic production of T_3 from T_4: deiodinases: the "guardians of the gate" to the nuclear T_3 receptors. *Top*: Local and systemic production of T_3 from T_4 contributing to the occupation of nuclear T_3 receptors and exported into the circulation, typical of the hepatocyte. *Middle*: Almost exclusive local production of T_3 contributing to the occupation of nuclear T_3 receptors, typical of the hypothyroid brain and pituitary. *Bottom*: Local and systemic production of T_3 from T_4 contributing to the occupation of nuclear T_3 receptors and exported into the circulation, typical of the thyrocyte

et al. 1991). These findings suggest that in the thyrocyte too, a tissue-specific location of 5′-DI has to be expected. It has to be remembered that despite the immense hydrophobicity of the iodinated diphenylether structure of iodothyronines, these hormones cannot easily permeate cellular membranes, due to the presence of two highly charged functional groups at the distal parts of the molecule, the zwitter-ionic double-charged alanine side chain and the strongly acidic 4′-phenol group, which dissociates even at neutral pH. The thyrocyte has even a more serious problem to solve in terms of cell biology. The route of thyroid hormone secretion after complete proteolysis of thyroglobulin (Tg) in the lysosomal compartment via the plasma membrane is a complete "black box". No evidence of ordered or regulated release of T_4 and/or T_3 from the thyroid cell is available, no specific T_4- and/or T_3-containing secretory vesicles have been seen in thyrocytes, and no specific regulation of the hormone secretion process by TSH, which controls nearly every step in thyroid hormone synthesis and secretion, has been described. One cannot imagine that T_4 and T_3, with the above-mentioned characteristics, easily permeate membranes. And if they did, the 5′-DI and the nuclear receptors would be continuously occupied, with the amount of thyroid hormones present in the thyrocyte under basal conditions and after TSH or TSAb stimulation. It has to be postulated that the thyrocyte has a unique system of thyroid hormone compartmentalization and a trafficking device similar to the highly ordered process of Tg synthesis and processing. Therefore it is surprising that no molecular defects involving lesions or alterations of thyroid hormone activation by the deiodinases have yet been found. Probably defects in 5′-DI expression and function are lethal (KÖHRLE 1983, 1994a) and therefore have not yet been described, in a similar way to the lack of viable mutations of the TRα nuclear T_3 receptor, although many TRβ mutants with different phenotype expression have now been found (REFETOFF et al. 1993).

Recently, in addition to the demonstration of thyroid-specific expression of thyroid hormone receptors (ERKENBRACK and ROSENBERG 1986; AKIGUCHI et al. 1992; DEGROOT et al. 1989; NAKAMURA and IMURA 1988), the presence of specific, high-affinity cytosolic thyroid hormone-binding proteins has been suggested in thyrocytes (ROUSSET, personal communucation). Probably these proteins are involved in reducing free thyroid hormone concentrations inside the thyrocytes and may contribute to controlled trafficking of hormones for deiodination, export for secretion, or import to the nuclear compartment for receptor activation. Apart from the 5′-DI, no other thyroid protein has been shown to be under the control of thyroid hormone, whether it be T_4 or T_3, "the chicken or the egg".

1.4 Drug Effects on Thyroid 5′-DI Activity and Thyroid Hormone Secretion

In addition to starvation, carbohydrate supply, several conditions related to the low-T_3 syndrome and non-thyroid illness (fever, post-trauma status, surgery, etc.) (HESCH 1981; KÖHRLE et al. 1991; KÖHRLE 1994a), thyroid T_3 production and secretion is also altered by several clinically administered or experimental drugs. Orally administered iodinated X-ray contrast agents such as ipodate, iopanoate and related compounds with iodinated aromatic or phenolic ring structures block 5′-DI and also thyroid hormone transport through plasma and intracellular membranes, and also compete for nuclear receptor binding of T_3 (LAURBERG 1982; CURRAN and DEGROOT 1991; GREEN 1991; KÖHRLE 1994b). The effect of these compounds generally leads to decreased circulating levels of T_3, accompanied by normal to elevated T_4 and generally elevated serum levels of rT_3. The increase of rT_3 is due to decreased rT_3-5′-deiodination in the liver and kidney resulting from inhibition of 5′-DI in these tissues, while the production of rT_3 in extrathyroid tissues expressing 5-deiodinase activity (e.g. brain, skin, placenta) is not affected by these agents. The exact contribution of decreased thyroid deiodination of T_4 to T_3 by these agents to the altered circulating thyroid hormone levels is not completely clear and is also different in different species. It has to be remembered that thyroid hormone economy and kinetics in the rat – the most frequently used experimental animal model for studying thyroid hormone regulation, synthesis, metabolism and action – differ considerably from those in the human. In the rat, TBG, the high-affinity binding protein for T_4, is only expressed in the neonatal and old animal and under conditions of carbohydrate overfeeding (YOUNG et al. 1982; VRANCKX et al. 1990). Due to the lack of this high-affinity serum transport and binding protein for T_4 (and T_3) the rat rapidly reaches hypothyroid conditions, leading to alterations of the hypothalamus, pituitary, thyroid and peripheral feedback system.

Nevertheless, those iodinated contrast agents have been tested as inhibitors of T_3 production and secretion during hyperthyroidism (WU et al. 1978; COSTA 1979; SHARP et al. 1981; BENG et al. 1980). However, the use of these agents for treatment of thyrotoxicosis, Graves' disease or iodine-induced hyperthyroidism should be avoided because the high iodine content of these compounds leads to severe and long-standing iodine contamination of the patient. These compounds are stored in the adipose tissue and slowly release iodide because they are weak substrates for all three iodothyronine deiodinase isozymes, and also for the enzymes degrading thyroid hormones by an oxidative, radical mechanism (e.g. the unspecific dehalogenases and enzymatic ether-ring cleavage) (KÖHRLE 1994a). Similar alterations of thyroid hormone metabolism are also found after administration of amiodarone, a widely used antiarrhythmic iodine-containing drug, which severely disturbs thyroid hormone secretion, deiodination, and action by a mechanism similar to the iodinated X-ray contrast agents (CURRAN and DEGROOT 1991; GREEN 1991; KÖHRLE 1994a). Administration of this drug should be avoided when ever possible, and precautionary measures such as a thorough evaluation of thyroid hormone status are mandatory before it is prescribed. (For a review of interference of other drugs with thyroid hormone status see CURRAN and DEGROOT 1991; GREEN 1991; KÖHRLE 1994a.) Recently, a series of experimental compounds have also been shown to interfere with T_3 production and secretion by the thyroid. A synthetic flavonoid, EMD 21388, known to be a potent inhibitor of 5′-DI and 5′-DII but also a selective and highly effective competitor of thyroid hormone binding to transthyretin (TTR, previously called thyroxine-binding prealbumin, TBPA), effectively increases thyroid T_3 production in the rat under conditions where the T_4 production rate and T_4 serum concentration are reduced and TSH serum levels are not increased (KÖHRLE et al. 1989; SCHRÖDER-VAN DER

Elst et al. 1991; Köhrle 1992, 1994a). The mechanism of action of this interesting compound on the thyroid is not known, and this implies that regulation of thyroid hormone production, deiodination and secretion is effectively controlled by several regulatory loops. In vitro, using thyroid cell lines or thyroid (cell) membrane preparations, EMD 21388 effectively inhibits 5′-DI, similar to findings in other tissues (Spanka et al. 1990; Köhrle 1992). The group of Gaitan reported that naturally occurring and widely consumed flavonoids (contained in millet and other goitrogenic, plant-derived nutrients) as well as some synthetic flavonoid compounds effectively block several steps in thyroid hormone synthesis and secretion (Gaitan et al. 1989). For this reason attention has to be paid to potential side effects of clinically used and experimental drugs showing structural similarity to thyroid hormones, i.e. most aromatic, phenolic mono- or polycyclic compounds with hydrophobic (iodinated X-ray contrast agents, amiodarone) or hydrophilic (flavonoids) properties.

1.5 Are There Direct Effects of T_4 on Thyroid Function?

Direct effects of T_4 on thyroid function or action have not been shown. In the brain, in rat astrocytes and brown adipose tissue of rodents, T_4 by itself, without being deiodinated to the thyromimetically active hormone T_3, has direct effects at the plasma membrane level (Leonard 1991). T_4 (and also rT_3, but not T_3) rapidly – in the minute range – promotes polymerization of the actin cytoskeleton. Independent of the actin polymerization process, which can also be stimulated by retinoids, a second direct effect of T_4 (and rT_3 but not T_3) occurs in rat astrocytes which has not been described in tissues or cells expressing type I 5′-D activity (Leonard 1991). T_4 rapidly inactivates the 5′-DII enzyme which is cytosolically orientated on the inner side of the plasma membrane (Safran et al. 1993). This process also requires an interaction between the polymerized F-actin, T_4 and the 5′-DII isozyme (Leonard 1991; Farwell et al. 1993; Safran et al. 1993; Farwell and Leonard 1992). This second direct T_4 effect might contribute to the brain-specific regulation of 5′-DII activity and local production of T_3 in these tissues which are independent of circulating plasma T_3, which is formed by the 5′-DI isozyme of thyroid, liver and kidney.

Rapid effects on the polymerization of the actin cytoskeleton have also been demonstrated for TSH, which rapidly depolymerized F-actin in dog thyrocytes in cell cultures (Roger et al. 1989; Demeure et al. 1990; Siegel 1976). Whether TSH effects on the thyrocyte actin cytoskeleton alter thyroid hormone deiodination, secretion or action in the thyroid itself remains to be studied.

1.6 Nuclear T_3 Receptors in Thyrocytes

Until recently, no clear evidence for direct effects of thyroid hormones on the human thyroid gland itself had been obtained. The feedback regulation of thyroid hormone synthesis, secretion, and action has been located in the hypothalamus, the anterior pituitary and the extrathyroid tissues which produce T_3 from T_4 by the 5′-DI isozyme (KÖHRLE 1994a). Controversial data have been reported concerning a direct inhibitory short-loop feedback of thyroid hormones on TSH stimulation (for review see NAKAMURA and IMURA 1988). Previously, thyroid hormone effects were determined by global parameters such as increased basal or thyroid hormone-stimulated metabolic rate and oxygen consumption or, later on, by studies of tracer binding to isolated nuclei or nuclear extracts containing T_3-binding sites. Due to the high endogenous thyroid hormone content in thyroid nuclei or nuclear extracts, no definitive data on thyroid hormone receptors have been established. Recently, with the improved characterization of the T_3 receptor proteins, availability of advanced T_3 binding and displacement assays and successful cloning of the c-erbA family of nuclear T_3 receptors, the presence of functional T_3 receptors in thyroid tissue and even their regulation by the thyroid hormone status has been unequivocally demonstrated (NAKAMURA and IMURA 1988; PISAREV et al. 1986; DEGROOT et al. 1989; ERKENBRACK and ROSENBERG 1986; AKIGUCHI et al. 1992; SELMI-RUBY and ROUSSET 1994; SAKURAI et al. 1989; KAMIKUBO et al. 1992). Thyroid tissue and cell lines express both the α- and β-forms of the T_3 receptor, which are not completely saturated by their ligand T_3. The functionality of these receptors has been demonstrated, for example, by the thyroid hormone-dependent regulation of 5′-DI expression and stimulation of malic enzyme (KOHN et al. 1989) and cell proliferation in FRTL-5 cells (AKIGUCHI et al. 1992). Whereas T_3 receptor numbers and mRNA levels are rather low in the rat FRTL-5 thyroid cell line, both very high receptor numbers and very high mRNA levels have been found in porcine and human thyroid tissue, at concentrations exceeding even those in liver (NAKAMURA and IMURA 1988; DEGROOT et al. 1989; SAKURAI et al. 1989; KAMIKUBO et al. 1992). Immunofluorescence studies also revealed a nuclear location of the TRβ-receptor in rat thyroid (DEGROOT et al. 1989), similar to the location in other tissues. In a transient transfection system of pig thyrocytes in primary culture, functional activity of endogenous thyrocyte T_3 receptors for stimulation of a T_3-responsive reporter gene could be shown (SELMI-RUBY and ROUSSET 1994). TSH had no effect on basal or T_3-stimulated activity of the TRE-driven reporter gene (SELMI-RUBY and ROUSSET 1994). At present it is unclear whether there exists a functional relationship between these high T_3 receptor numbers and the highest specific activities determined for 5′-DI in thyroid tissue. With the unequivocal identification of T_3 receptors in human, dog and rat thyroid tissue, the existence of autocrine or short-loop feedback mechanisms of regulation of thyroid function and secretion by thyroid hormones has to be considered, especially in the gland hyperstimulated by TSH or thyroid-stimulating antibodies (TSAb) or in thyroid cancer tissue (see below).

Tissue-specific expression, receptor number, binding capacity, saturation and functional activity of T_3 receptors is altered by many patho-physiological conditions such as thyroid state, starvation, the low-T_3 syndrome, diabetes and uraemia (OPPENHEIMER et al. 1987; DEGROOT et al. 1989; CHIN et al. 1993; HESCH 1981; WARTOFSKY and BURMAN 1993; YEN and CHIN 1994). The role of thyroid function, secretory activity and T_3/T_4 secretion ratio under these conditions is still a matter of controversy. The identification of TRβ-receptor mutants, in vitro and in vivo expression or "knockout" of the different receptor forms or their mutants in thyroid cells or transgenic animals will provide detailed information on their role in thyroid function.

1.7 Role of the Trace Elements Iodine and Selenium in Thyroid Hormone Deiodination in the Thyroid Gland

Iodine is one of the two trace elements essential for thyroid hormone synthesis and proper thyroid function. The evolution of the thyroid gland is an unique example of how specialization of a specific tissue can guarantee continuous supply of this highly essential trace element for thyroid hormone synthesis even in species living outside marine habitats; these elements have been washed out from the territory and soil in most areas of the populated world. So far no direct effects of iodide on thyroid 5′-DI expression and T_3 receptor levels have been demonstrated. However, iodine deficiency leads to decreased iodination of Tg and to enhanced TSH stimulation after long-term serious iodine deficiency (Medeiros-Neto et al. 1993; Brabant et al. 1992). Therefore, indirect stimulatory effects mediated via the TSH-signal transduction pathways have to be expected for 5′-DI activity and probably also the T_3 receptor expression. In contrast to the stimulation of cell growth by T_3, no direct effect of T_3 could be shown in vitro in the FRTL-5 cell model on iodide uptake and basal or TSH-stimulated cAMP-production, whereas TSH-stimulated increase of iodide uptake was slightly inhibited by nanomolar T_3 concentrations (Akiguchi et al. 1992).

Very recently, the essential role of a second trace element, selenium, for thyroid hormone synthesis, metabolism and action has been recognized (Köhrle 1994a; Contempre et al. 1991a). While it had already been postulated that selenium had a part in thyroid hormone synthesis and thyroid function, a major breakthrough in understanding thyroid hormone metabolism was achieved in 1990 with the identification of 5′-DI as the second eukaryotic selenoprotein with a known enzyme function (Behne et al. 1990; Arthur et al. 1990). Biochemical characterization followed by cloning of the 5′-DI cDNA clearly identified the presence of selenocysteine, a rare amino acid in the active site of 5′-DI in thyroid, liver, kidney and other tissues (Behne et al. 1990; Arthur et al. 1990; Berry et al. 1991; Safran et al. 1991). In contrast to 5′-DI, the 5′-DII isozyme and 5-deiodinase are not selenoenzymes (Köhrle 1994a; Safran et al. 1991).

The selenoprotein nature of 5′-DI also allows us to understand the pathogenesis of the myxoedematous form of endemic cretinism, which is still prevalent in many parts of the world (Contempre et al. 1991a,b). While the neurological form of endemic cretinism can probably be explained by the exclusive lack of iodine, the myxoedematous form originates under conditions of combined iodine and selenium deficiency. The lack of selenium seems to protect the fetus from thyroid hormone deficiency during pregnancy due to the lack of expression of 5′-DI which accounts for deiodination of T_4 and elimination of T_4, T_3 and other thyroid hormone metabolites, a process combined with urinary loss of iodide (Contempre et al. 1991a,b; KÖHRLE 1994a). Apparently 5′-DII in the fetal brain (and other tissues) provides enough locally produced T_3 to prevent neurological damage during fetal development, when the maternal organism contributes at least minimal amounts of thyroid hormone for the fetus. After birth, the baby then slowly reaches the condition of thyroid hormone deficiency, because continuous stimulation of the thyroid by TSH under these conditions generates massive amounts of H_2O_2 and oxygen radicals which cannot be used or degraded in the newborn thyroid for two reasons: firstly, the lack of iodine and a substrate for the iodination and coupling reaction of Tg catalyzed by TPO does not consume H_2O_2 and oxygen radicals; secondly, the normal thyroid gland is known to contain selenium concentrations higher than kidney and some other endocrine organs (for review see KÖHRLE 1994a, 1995). The high concentration of selenium in the thyroid is partially due to high concentrations of glutathione peroxidase (GPx), the first identified eukaryotic selenoenzyme (and possibly also due to the high 5′-DI activity). It is known that GPx (and catalase) are involved in destruction of toxic H_2O_2 and other oxygen radicals and that expression of GPx depends strictly on selenium supply. Under conditions of selenium deficiency, thyroid GPx activity might also be decreased (like the serum and liver enzyme), thus fuelling into the fatal circle of enhanced H_2O_2 and oxygen radical production, concomitant to decreased consumption and degradation, with the long-term result of complete destruction of thyroid tissue, which is observed in myxoedematous endemic cretinism (CONTEMPRE et al. 1991a,b). This concept of the pathogenesis of myxoedematous cretinism has been supported by a trial attempting to prevent this disease by supplementation with iodine, selenium or both trace elements. The trial was stopped immediately after it turned out that selenium supplementation without previous sufficient restoration of iodine stores rapidly leads to elimination and degradation of the residual low amounts of circulating thyroid hormone (CONTEMPRE et al. 1991b). This probably occurs by a rapid selenium-dependent restoration of 5′-DI activity which forms T_3 and degrades other iodothyronines (KÖHRLE 1994a) under conditions where iodine liberated as product of the reaction cannot be either recovered or utilized for new hormone synthesis in the damaged gland. Apparently, under conditions of selenium deficiency, restoration of 5′-DI by selenium occurs preferentially before GPx activity is restored (GROSS et al. 1992, 1994; OERTEL et al. 1993). This cellular hierarchy of preferential selenium supply for 5′-DI over GPx is overlaid by a tissue hierarchy of selenium supply under conditions of deficiency: while muscle, liver and kidney lose selenium (and 5′-DI activity), selenium seems to be retained or even redistributed to certain endocrine organs (testes, thyroid, adrenals) and to the brain (BEHNE et al. 1988; BURK et al. 1972). However, it is remarkable in this context that even during severe experimental selenium depletion of the rat, thyroid 5′-DI activity is still maintained at roughly normal levels, while 5′-DI of liver and kidney are severely decreased or lost (MEINHOLD et al. 1993; CHANOINE et al. 1993). It might be speculated that maintenance of intrathyroid T_3 production from T_4 is extremely critical to residual thyroid function even under these severe pathological conditions. These latter findings further indicate the essential role of 5′-DI in thyroid and brain function.

1.8 Peculiar Properties of Thyrocytes from Different Species: The Pig Model

Freshly isolated pig thyrocytes and primary cultures of pig thyroid exhibit several peculiarities compared to model systems using thyrocytes from other species. Firstly, pig thyroids show a high saturation by iodide, probably because pigs receive a high iodine supply with their fodder (R. GÄRTNER, personal communication). Secondly, pig thyroid tissue shows different response to TSH and other growth factors than do dog, rat and human thyroid, i.e. TSH does not directly stimulate pig thyrocyte growth on its own, but only via TSH-induced auto- and paracrine factors (GORETZKI et al. 1990; DUMONT et al. 1992; VASSART and DUMONT 1992; GÄRTNER et al. 1990). Thirdly, expression of functional 5′-DI is surprisingly low in the thyroid tissue and cells of the "omnivorous" pig (similar to the herbivores) compared to other omnivores such as man, rodents, and guinea pigs (BEECH et al. 1993). This finding relates not only to enzyme activity: we could not even detect steady-state mRNA levels by Northern blotting analysis or reverse transcriptase polymerase chain reaction using primer pairs complementary to the rat or human 5′-DI sequence (unpublished data). Fourthly, freshly isolated pig thyrocytes contain unusually high (free?) thyroid hormone concentrations (NISHIDA et al. 1991). This last finding sugggests a powerful retention mechanism or expression of high-affinity and/or high-capacity binding proteins for both T_4 and T_3, because Tg could not be demonstrated in the porcine follicular cells in monolayer culture. The peculiar functional consequences of these observations are not clear, but have to be borne in mind when porcine thyroid cells are used as a model.

1.9 Alterations of 5′-DI and T_3 Receptor Expression in Human Thyroid Carcinoma Tissues and Cell Lines

While 5′-DI and nuclear T_3 receptors are highly abundant in normal thyroid tissues of several species and differentiated thyroid cell lines, marked alterations of the expression and function of both 5′-DI and T_3 receptors are found during the process of dedifferentiation of the thyroid gland to thyroid carcinoma and also in cultured thyroid carcinoma cell lines. As mentioned above, expression of 5′-DI and its 27-kDa substrate binding subunit is elevated in thyroid tissue from patients with Graves' disease and also in thyroid adenoma (KÖHRLE et al. 1993; TOYODA et al. 1990, 1992b; SUGAWARA et al. 1984; KÖHRLE 1994a). Analysing a series of differentiated and anaplastic thyroid carcinoma, we found marked alterations of expression of 5′-DI activity and its 27-kDa substrate binding subunit (KÖHRLE et al. 1993, 1994). As in normal tissues and cell lines, 5′-DI activity and the abundance of its substrate binding subunit are always in parallel, which is compatible with the ideas that 5′-DI is a homodimer, that the subunit alone is devoid of activity and that no post-translational modification of the 5′-DI enzyme has yet been described (KÖHRLE 1994a). Compared to "normal" thyroid tissue (tissue surrounding the tumour, or parts of the gland removed during resection of parathyroid adenoma),

5′-DI activity and expression of the subunit in differentiated follicular thyroid carcinoma were found to be decreased and in dedifferentiated anaplastic carcinoma tissue they were very low to undetectable. In papillary thyroid carcinoma, low to normal but also in some few cases highly elevated 5′-DI activity was determined. Expression of 5′-DI did not directly correlate to other thyroid-specific differentiation markers such as TSH receptor, Tg or TPO (Köhrle et al. 1993, 1994). Decreased 5′-DI expression was also found in five cases of papillary adenocarcinoma by another group (Toyoda et al. 1992b). Our results are compatible with the current model of the pathogenetic events leading to thyroid carcinoma, which suggests that papillary thyroid carcinoma is initiated by mechanisms different from that give rise to follicular thyroid carcinoma, but that both forms can eventually lead to the anaplastic form of thyroid cancer (Wynford-Thomas 1993; Herrmann et al. 1991; Farid et al. 1994).

In order to confirm these findings, experiments were initiated using several human thyroid carcinoma cell lines for analysis of 5′-DI expression and its regulation in thyroid tissue. As expected from the analysis of anaplastic carcinoma tissues, no 5′-DI (nor 5′-DII) activity was detectable in the two human anaplastic thyroid carcinoma cell lines HTh 74 and C 643 available for our studies (Schreck et al. 1994; Köhrle et al. 1993). Neither did variation of culture conditions (e.g. removal of serum, addition of growth factors and hormones) induce 5′-DI expression. So far no papillary carcinoma cell line has been available to us. In two follicular thyroid carcinoma cell lines (FTC-133 and FTC-238) derived from the same patient, very low basal 5′-DI activities could be determined, about three orders of magnitude below those of the differentiated rat FRTL-5 cells (Schreck et al. 1994; Oertel et al. 1991). These FTC cells express low numbers of functional TSH receptors, secrete small amounts of Tg into the medium, but already show a dedifferentiated morphology (Goretzki et al. 1990; Goretzki 1996; Demeure et al. 1992). Transplantation of FTC-133 cells onto athymic nude rats, which exhibit a reduced immune response to xenotransplants, confirmed that the low basal expression of 5′-DI in FTC cells, which grow to solid tumours on these rats, is an endogenous property of these cells and not dependent on cell culture conditions (Hoang-Vu et al. 1992b; Köhrle et al. 1993). In four of six tumours grown after xenotransplantation, a very low but measurable 5′-DI activity was shown; in the two other tumours 5′-DI activity was at or below the detection limit (M. Oertel, C. Hoang-Vu, J. Köhrle, unpublished data). Like the results obtained under cell culture conditions, these two tumours were positive for Tg in immunohistochemical analysis, and it was even possible to monitor growth of the tumour by serum determination of human Tg by a specific Tg immuno-radiometric assay (IRMA) which does not detect endogenous rat Tg (Hoang-Vu et al. 1992b). After retinoic acid treatment, xenotransplantation of the treated FTC cells led to significantly reduced tumour growth of the xenotransplanted cells, suggesting retinoid-induced alteration of the proliferation capacity of these partially "re-differentiated" human follicular thyroid carcinoma cells (M. Oertel, C. Hoang-Vu, J. Köhrle, unpublished data). Future studies will show whether other thyroid and tumour-specific differentiation markers are altered after retinoid-induced stimulation of 5′-DI activity in these cells, leading later to decreased proliferative, invasive and metastatic potential.

1.10 Retinoids Induce 5′-DI Expression in Follicular Thyroid Carcinoma Cells

In order to test our hypothesis that 5′-DI expression is lost during the process of dedifferentiation of thyrocytes via follicular to anaplastic carcinoma, we tried to re-differentiate these follicular thyroid carcinoma lines in the direction of normal thyrocytes (SCHRECK et al. 1994). Retinoids are known to be potent inducers of differentiation and morphogenesis and are clinically used in the (re-)differentiation therapy of acute promyelocytic leukaemia and also of solid epithelial tumours. A single application of nanomolar concentrations of all-*trans*-retinoic acid and also of other retinoids to cultured FTC cells in the absence or presence of serum leads to rapid and marked induction of 5′-DI in these cell lines, whereas no such effect was obtained in the two anaplastic thyroid carcinoma lines. Stimulation of 5′-DI activity and expression of its 27-kDa substrate binding subunit reached a plateau after 2–3 days and was maintained at this level for several days. Inhibitors of transcription and translation blocked this retinoid-induced 5′-DI stimulation. Thyroid hormones were unable to mimic this retinoid effect and did not enhance retinoid stimulation if added together with retinoids. No such retinoid effect was observed in the differentiated rat FRTL-5 cells, where 5′-DI activity was already expressed at levels similar to those in normal thyroid tissue. As a control, the retinoid effect was also determined for alkaline phosphatase, a retinoid-sensitive differentiation marker of various epithelial and stem cells. Alkaline phosphatase was stimulated by retinoids in all four thyroid cells lines to various degrees and, again, the already differentiated FRTL-5 cells expressed high basal levels of alkaline phosphatase which were no further stimulated by retinoids. The latter findings suggest that the retinoid signal transduction pathway is still intact even in anaplastic thyroid cell lines, Furthermore, the stimulatory effect of retinoids on 5′-DI is restricted to follicular thyroid carcinoma lines, indicating that the two anaplastic carcinoma lines have reached a "point of no return" with respect to 5′-DI expression, due to mutations and defects related to the tumour initiation, promotion and de-differentiation processes (SCHRECK et al. 1994). Decrease or loss of 5′-DI expression has also been found in human kidney cancer (NAUMANN et al. 1993), suggesting that the capacity for cellular T_3 production in certain epithelial cells that express 5′-DI activity under normal conditions is essential for normal cellular function. Further results compatible with the loss of 5′-DI expression are immunohistochemical findings in 62 specimens of metastases of differentiated thyroid carcinoma, where T_4 and Tg immunoreactivity was observed in 60 specimens but positive T_3 signals in only 4 of the whole 62 (BÄTGE et al. 1992).

In a recent study using intact porcine thyroid follicles in culture after initial embedding in a collagen matrix, 10 μM all-*trans*-retinoic acid reversibly decreased total T_4 and T_3 secretion into the culture medium compared to the normal control in the presence of a six-hormone mixture (HISHINUMA et al. 1992). However, if one calculates the T_3/T_4 ratio secreted by these cells during the whole 12-day treatment period, a clear decrease from 0.57 (days 0–4) to 0.47 (days 5–8) to 0.41 (days 9–12), or a T_3/T_4 ratio of 0.47 (total hormone secreted), is seen in the control group, while in the retinoic acid group the starting ratio of 0.59 is maintained over the whole period (0.55: days 5–8; 0.63: days 9–12; 0.58: total hormone secreted). We interpret these published data as evidence for retinoic acid-regulated maintenance of 5′-DI expression. Alteration of the iodination ratio of Tg is less probable because the authors performed their studies in the presence of 0.1 μM NaI, which should supply enough iodide for efficient hormone synthesis in culture. However, retinoids in culture reduce iodine uptake, TSH-stimulated TPO and Tg expression and TSH-stimulated organification in vitro in porcine thyroid culture models (NAMBA et al. 1993) and also in one human follicular thyroid carcinoma line (VAN HERLE et al. 1990), which expresses a very low deiodinase activity with characteristics discordant from those found in our experiments using the FTC-133 and FTC-238 lines (SCHRECK et al. 1994).

1.11 Does Expression of 5′-DI in Human Thyroid Cancer or Its Metastases Lead to Alterations of the Thyroid Status?

Reports on the prevalence of concurrent or previous hyperthyroidism due to thyroid cancer or its metastasis are very rare despite the potential for iodide concentration, hormone synthesis, metabolism and secretion in many tumours or their metastases. In a study of 502 thyroid cancer patients, only 10 were found to be hyperthyroid due to Graves' disease, multinodular goitre, nodules or large functional tumour (for review see EDMONDS and TELLEZ 1988; SARDA et al. 1989; SUNG and CAVALIERI 1973; OTTEVANGER et al. 1992). A few rare cases of T_3 thyrotoxicosis due to metastatic follicular thyroid carcinoma after removal of the primary tumour were reported, but no data on 5′-DI activity in these tumours were available. It is therefore not possible to discriminate between enhanced T_3 production via 5′-deiodination of T_4 or a defect in the iodination of Tg omitting the T_4 coupling sites and using only the T_3 hormonogenic site (for review see MEDEIROS-NETO et al. 1993). However, the review by PAUL and SISSON (1990) mentions that half of the 48 patients presented with elevated T_3 and normal or low T_4 serum thyroid hormone levels, while the remainder had elevations of both hormones. The frequency of thyroid carcinoma in hyperthyroidism and Graves' disease is still a matter of controversy (for reviews see SARDA et al. 1989; PAUL and SISSON 1990; MAZZAFERRI 1990; HALES et al. 1992).

1.12 Role of TSH-Suppressive T_4 Therapy for T_3 Production by 5′-DI in Thyroid Carcinoma

The current concept of TSH-suppressive therapy of thyroid cancer by T_4 is based on the assumption that suppression of TSH leads to reduced thyroid and tumour growth stimulation (BURMEISTER et al. 1992). The limitations of this therapy need to be discussed under two headings. Firstly, many thyroid carcinomas no longer express functional TSH receptors, so endogenous TSH cannot exert a growth stimulatory effect (BRABANT et al. 1991; HOANG-VU et al. 1992a, 1993; SHI et al.

1993; Elisei et al. 1994), and therefore no growth stimulation will be mediated via the TSH/TSH-receptor signalling pathway. Impairment of the TSH G-protein signal transduction system has been reported in human thyroid carcinoma cells (Kimura et al. 1922b). Secondly, the demonstration of high activity of 5′-DI in normal thyrocytes and some papillary thyroid carcinomas and low but measurable 5′-DI activity in follicular thyroid carcinoma and a few anaplastic carcinomas raises the question of growth stimulation by T_3 formed in these cells via 5′-DI (Köhrle et al. 1993; Schreck et al. 1994). It has been reported in some animal models and in epidemiological studies that T_3 stimulates tumour initiation, maintenance, growth, proliferation and metastatic potential (Kumar et al. 1979; Short and Ove 1983; Borek et al. 1983; Leuthauser and Guernsey 1987; Lopez et al. 1989; Sellitti et al. 1981). Although these data are somewhat controversial, attention has to be paid to a potentially negative effect of TSH-suppressive T_4 therapy, which might lead to increased T_3 production in the tumour or its metastases. On the other hand, several studies show the essential role of T_3 for cell differentiation. Therefore, a final conclusion about whether 5′-DI-mediated T_3 production plays a beneficial or a deleterious role in thyroid carcinoma cannot be drawn yet. Coordinated interaction between retinoids and T_3 via their nuclear receptors might be a prerequisite for maintenance of a differentiated epithelial thyrocyte function, similar to the requirement for continuous regulation for differentiation in general. The loss of 5′-DI expression and tightly controlled local T_3 production during the process of de-differentiation of thyroid carcinoma could be one of the molecular defects of growth control leading to loss of growth control and increased tendency for invasion and metastasis (Schreck et al. 1994). Another consequence of the frequently increased T_3/T_4 ratio might be that it becomes necessary to determine both T_3 and T_4 serum levels in thyroid cancer patients. The age and sex distribution of patients with differentiated thyroid carcinoma causing thyrotoxicosis are no different from those of patients with euthyroid thyroid carcinoma.

2 Thyroid Differentiation Markers and Thyroid Carcinoma

2.1 Irradiation and Thyroid Cancer

"Thyroid cancer is one of the most sensitive indicators of childhood radiation exposure" (Schneider et al. 1993; see also for current update and review Wynford-Thomas 1993; Schneider et al. 1993; Franceschi et al. 1993; Clark and Duh 1990; DeGroot 1993; Ron et al. 1994; Langsteger et al. 1993). Recently the issue of radiation-induced thyroid cancer has attracted tremendous interest after various reports of a highly increased incidence (more than ten-fold) of an unusual form of childhood thyroid cancer in areas with high fallout after the Chernobyl nuclear accident (Baverstock et al. 1992; Kazakov et al. 1992; Ron et al. 1992; Williams 1993; EORTC Thyroid Study Group Meeting 1993, Cardiff, UK). The increased incidence in children in this area of papillary carcinomas with a strong tendency to invasiveness raised the issue of differences in the aetiology and the molecular events of tumour initiation, promotion, proliferation, invasiveness and metastatic tendency (WYNFORD-THOMAS 1993; FRANCESCHI et al. 1993; WILLIAMS 1993). So far we have no clear picture of why different forms of thyroid carcinoma behave differently as to tumour progression, invasiveness and metastasis. Earlier epidemiological and neck radiation follow-up studies revealed that the risk of thyroid carcinoma increased with the radiation dose (SCHNEIDER et al. 1993; ITO et al. 1986).

2.2 Loss, Expression and Overexpression of Oncogenes and Thyroid-Specific Genes in Thyroid Carcinoma

A series of molecular defects have been described which either occur in all types of thyroid carcinomas or are only found with some prevalence in the different varieties. This subject has been extensively covered in several recent reviews, and models for the different pathogenetic events in the development of thyroid carcinoma have been put forward on the basis of the description of molecular defects, their consequences, and results of epidemiological, retrospective or prospective clinical studies (WYNFORD-THOMAS 1993; WYLLIE et al. 1989; FRANCESCHI et al. 1993; GRIECO et al. 1990; HERRMANN et al. 1991; LEMOINE et al. 1988; FRANCIS LANG et al. 1992; HASHIMOTO et al. 1990). Among several proto-oncogenes or their mutated variants, the classical nuclear c-myc, N-myc, c-fos, c-erbA family, the cytosolic ras family, receptor-type oncogenes, and thyrocyte-specific gene rearrangements (ret) or loss of heterozygosity with evidence of a loss of tumour suppressor genes have been found to be altered or involved in the pathogenic sequence (WYNFORD-THOMAS 1993; FRANCESCHI et al. 1993; GRIECO et al. 1990; HERRMANN et al. 1991; LEMOINE et al. 1988).

Many papillary thyroid carcinomas seem to originate in a translocation of the ret oncogene, coding for a *re*ceptor *t*yrosine kinase to an as yet unknown aminoterminal sequence H4 (GRIECO et al. 1990). This translocation leads to detectable transcripts in papillary thyroid carcinoma and their metastases, but no activation of this oncogene, also called PTC, is found in follicular carcinoma (GRIECO et al. 1988, 1990; SANTORO et al. 1993; SUAREZ et al. 1991). It is interesting that point mutations in "hot spots" of the ret oncogene on human chromosome 10 are apparently the cause of thyroid C cell carcinoma in MEN-2A (MULLIGAN et al. 1993). Low expression of the normal ret proto-oncogene is found in normal human thyroid tissue (SANTORO 1990). A recent report suggested that in vitro irradiation of thyroid and other cells leads to ret-PTC oncogene rearrangements similar to those found in papillary thyroid carcinoma, raising the possibility that irradiation is one of the major events in the pathogenic sequence leading to papillary thyroid carcinoma, the form of thyroid cancer predominant among Japanese atomic bomb survivors and children in the fallout area of the Chernobyl nuclear reactor catastrophe (ITO et al. 1993). Expression and activation of a second oncogene of the members of the tyrosine kinase receptor gene family, trk, has also been found in thyroid carcinoma (SANTORO et al. 1993; BONGARZONE et al. 1989). Several cytogenetic, clonal abnormalities, including loss of heterozygosity, were detected in papillary thyroid carcinoma, but also in follicular carcinoma (Herrmann et al. 1991; Matsuo et al. 1991), especially on chromosomes 3p, 10q, an 11q13; some of these findings were not confirmed, however. Aberrant DNA methylation patterns were also described for human thyroid carcinoma, which might contribute to cell transformation in the early stages of thyroid tumour formation (Matsuo et al. 1993b). In papillary carcinoma, overexpression or accumulation of the tumour suppressor gene p53 is also found (Zou et al. 1993). Mutations in this gene markedly prolong the half-life of this otherwise very short-lived protein. However, controversial evidence of p53 mutations has been presented for thyroid carcinoma in contrast to thyroid carcinoma cell lines (Ain et al. 1992; Goretzki 1993; Zou et al. 1993; Wright et al. 1989). The increased levels of this mutated p53 protein in papillary thyroid carcinoma easily allow its detection by immunohistochemistry. However, it remains unclear why increased levels of a tumour suppressor gene without identified mutations are found in cancer tissue (Wynford-Thomas 1993; Dockhorn-Dwonrniczak et al. 1993). It might be speculated that this is an event secondary to the primary cause of tumour initiation, growth, or proliferation, because the lesioned cells are trying everything to suppress tumour growth, and this might involve among other things increased expression of p53 or its mutant proteins. Mutated p53 has also been found in the follicular thyroid carcinoma cell lines FTC-133 and FTC-238, and accumulation of the p53 protein has been shown by immunohistochemistry in nuclei of these cells in cultures (Simon et al. 1993), where growth arrest by bleomycin does not work any more and the p53 activation pathway is no longer functional (Bombick et al. 1988; Wynford-Thomas 1993).

TSH receptor mutations which lead to TSH-independent, constitutive activation of the adenylate cyclase are found in 30% of autonomously functioning thyroid adenoma (Parma et al. 1993), but have not been identified yet in thyroid carcinoma (Matsuo et al. 1993a). Impairment of TSH signal transduction was found in human thyroid carcinoma cells (Kimura et al. 1992b) and expression of the TSH receptor in conjunction with low expression of c-myc mRNA has been suggested to be associated with a good prognosis in thyroid carcinoma (Shi et al. 1993). However, more than 30% of thyroid carcinomas show mutations of the Gsα-protein (Goretzki et al. 1993; Matsuo et al. 1993a; O'Sullivan et al. 1991; Suarez et al. 1991), which couples the TSH receptor to the adenylate cyclase. Increased expression of the Gsα-protein was also demonstrated by immunohistochemistry (Derwahl et al. 1993). Probably mutations and (over-)expression of mutated Gsα-proteins are late and not primary events in thyroid carcinogenesis.

In 20% of papillary carcinomas (activating) ras mutations were found, which seem to be a late event in tumour proliferation (Namba et al. 1990a,b; Rochefort et al. 1993). Transgenic mice carrying ras mutations do not develop thyroid carcinoma, but only thyroid hyperplasia and lung nodules, which findings support the idea that *ras* mutations in thyroid carcinoma are secondary events contributing to tumour proliferation but not per se essential for the development of neoplasia (Rochefort et al. 1993). However, contradictory data on the expression of activating mutations of the various ras oncogenes have also been presented (Lemoine et al. 1988; SUAREZ et al. 1988, 1990; SCHMID 1993; NAMBA et al. 1990a; BASOLO et al. 1994; SANTORO et al. 1993; FRANCIS LANG et al. 1992).

More than 50% of papillary thyroid carcinoma overexpress the Met receptor, which uses hepatocyte growth factor (HGF) and "scatter factor" as ligands. Expression of the Met receptor is not specific to thyroid carcinoma and its functional role in thyroid carcinoma is as yet unclear (DI RENZO et al. 1991, 1992). Expression of Met receptor has not been observed in normal thyroid and benign thyroid adenoma (DI RENZO et al. 1991, 1992).

Follicular carcinomas have been shown to express the thyroid-specific transcription factors TTF-1 and TTF-2 (LAZZARO et al. 1991), and also PAX-8, another transcription factor essential in thyroid-specific gene expression. Transfection experiments revealed that (co-)expression of TTF-1 and PAX-8 is necessary but not sufficient for thyroid-specific expression of genes (LAZZARO et al. 1991).

c-myc is expressed in benign and malignant tumours as shown by in situ hybridization analysis (SCHMID 1993). Mutations of H-ras were found in thyroid neoplasms but not in normal tissues (NAMBA et al. 1990a,b).

Transfection of the epithelial thyroid cell line PC C1 3 of Fisher rat origin with E1A, the adenovirus gene coding for transcription activating nuclear proteins, lead to the combined loss of TSH-dependent growth, ability to trap iodide and synthesis of Tg, but no typical markers of neoplasia were observed (BERLINGIERI et al. 1993).

2.3 Cytokines, Growth Factors and Receptors in Thyroid Carcinoma

Normal human follicular cells in primary culture produce IL-8 among other cytokines (WEETMAN et al. 1992). While normal thyroid tissues express only low amounts of growth factors of the IGF and EGF families and their receptors, thyroid adenoma and carcinoma show much higher levels of these factors, most of which are produced in an auto- and/or paracrine fashion in the thyroid tissue (GÄRTNER 1993; EGGO and SHEPPARD 1994; MIYAMOTO et al. 1988). TGFα, which is activated by an elastase enzyme, is also expressed at higher levels in thyroid carcinoma and acts via the EGF receptor. It is still unclear whether these alterations in the expression and function of growth factors and their receptors in thyroid carcinoma are primary or secondary events of the complex processes of tumorigenesis and proliferation. In particular, the interaction between thyrocytes, endothelial cells, fibroblasts and the immune system in thyroid neoplasia is far from understood. In vitro, IL-1 secreted in an autocrine fashion was shown to inhibit human thyroid carcinoma cell growth (KIMURA et al. 1992a; ZEKI et al. 1993) in a similar way to somatostatin (AIN and TAYLOR 1994).

Elevated co-expression of the c-erbB2/neu and c-erbB oncogenes, receptors for EGF and related growth factors was demonstrated in papillary carcinoma and lymph node metastases (AASLAND et al. 1988), but again this may be a secondary event.

2.4 Cytoskeleton and Cell Adhesion Proteins in Thyroid Cancer

The invasiveness and metastatic tendency of differentiated thyroid carcinoma are apparently in inverse correlation to the expression of E-cadherin in the carcinoma tissue, as in breast cancer and other epithelial cancer cell lines (Brabant et al. 1993; Hoang-Vu et al. 1993; Takeichi 1993). E-cadherin might be involved in Ca^{2+}-regulated cell-cell adhesion in conjunction with integrins. Furthermore, in Hürthle cell carcinomata, aberrant cytosolic expression of E-cadherin was also found; normally E-cadherin is strictly located on the outer surface of the basolateral membrane (Brabant et al. 1993). In the latter study a correlation between the expression of a variant of the cluster of differentiation molecule CD44v on the thyrocyte cell surface and the metastatic tendency of the carcinoma was also observed. Antibodies generated against peptides of the exon 6 variant sequence recognize increased expression of this protein in thyroid adenoma and carcinoma, but show no signal in normal thyroid tissue. Together with E-cadherin, CD44v might be a very useful prognostic marker of the invasiveness and metastatic tendency of thyroid carcinoma.

In a series of cultured FTC cells (FTC-133, FTC-236, FTC-238) and subclones, an increased tendency for invasiveness correlated with increased synthesis and expression of β_1-integrins (a family of receptors for basal membrane and extracellular matrix components) and combined activation and secretion of (tumor-specific?) proteases which degrade extracellular matrix and basal membranes (Demeure et al. 1992).

In anaplastic thyroid carcinoma, co-expression of cytokeratins and vimentin was observed, which is not seen in normal epithelial cells (Schmid 1993). Expression of cytokeratins, especially keratin 19, might help to distinguish papillary thyroid carcinoma (all specimens were found positive for keratin 19) from follicular carcinoma and follicular adenoma (Schelfhout et al. 1989).

2.5 Environmental Factors and Nutrition

Epidemiological studies in countries with varying iodine supplies suggest that geographic and nutritional factors such as iodine consumption also affect the pattern of pathogenesis and the incidence of different thyroid tumors. In Japan, a country with a rich iodine supply – up to ten-fold higher than recommended – due to high consumption of sea-fish, seafood, and seaweeds, the relatively higher incidence of papillary thyroid carcinoma suggests that iodine may play an aetiological role in thyroid tumorigenesis (Ezaki et al. 1992) (for reviews see Wynford-Thomas 1993; Farid et al. 1994; Franceschi et al. 1993). Follicular carcinoma, prevalent in iodine-deficient regions with endemic goitre, and anaplastic thyroid carcinoma are less prevalent in Japan. In addition, Japan has a higher incidence than other countries of occult thyroid microcarcinoma, usually papillary, detected post mortem. The prevalence of tumours among women in Japan is similar to that in other countries (Reinwein et al. 1989).

An interrelationship between thyroid status, thyroid cancer and environmental toxins such as dioxins, polychorinated biphenyls, polychlorinated phenols, etc. has repeatedly been reported, but clear causal relationships are still rare (Barsano 1981; McKinney et al. 1985; McKinney 1985; Ito et al. 1986; Byrne et al. 1987; Pesatori et al. 1993). Halogenated polycyclic hydrocarbons and related compounds specifically interact with the thyroid hormone serum binding protein transthyretin (formerly called thyroxine-binding prealbumin) and displace T_4 from its binding site (Cody 1985; McKinney et al. 1985; McKinney 1985), but no direct interaction with or binding to the nuclear T_3-receptor was shown in vivo. The dioxin TCCD increases the expression of nuclear receptors of the c-erbA family in certain mice strains (Bombick et al. 1988). The toxicity of these environmental agents has been correlated to the thyroid status (Bastomsky 1974; Barsano 1981). An interaction between thyroid hormones and the cellular binding proteins for halogenated biphenyls and the Ah receptor components was also found (Buff and Bründl 1992). Nevertheless, the altered thyroid hormone synthesis and metabolism in connection with the structural and functional alterations caused by the carcinomatous thyroid gland are not yet understood (Collins and Capen 1980).

Acknowledgments. This work was supported in parts by grants from the Land Niedersachsen, the Deutsche Forschungsgemeinschaft (Wi 231/9-1, TP1), and the European Community (ERB SC1 *CT92-0831 and BMH1-CT92-0081). The skillful assistance of Mrs. D. Quack during preparation of this manuscript is gratefully acknowledged.

Note Added in Proof: In the meanwhile the type I and type II 5′-deiodinase and the 5-deiodinase (type III) were cloned and all three are selenoproteins. The promoter of the type I 5′-deiodinase contains two thyroid hormone responsive elements.

References

Aasland R, Lillehaug JR, Male R, Josedal O, Varhaug JE, Kleppe K (1988) Expression of oncogenes in thyroid tumours: coexpression of c-erbB2/neu and c-erbB. Br J Cancer 57: 358–363

Ain KB, Taylor KD (1994) Somatostatin analogs affect proliferation of human thyroid carcinoma cell lines in vitro. J Clin Endocrinol Metab 78: 1097–1102

Ain KB, Taylor KD, Banks ER, Pettigrew AL (1992) Characterization of an immortalized cell-line (KAK-1) from a benign human thyroid follicular adenoma. Thyroid 2: S49

Akiguchi I, Strauss K, Borges M, Silva JE, Moses AC (1992) Thyroid hormone receptors and 3,5,3′-triiodothyronine biological effects in FRTL5 thyroid follicular cells. Endocrinology 131: 1279–1287

Arthur JR, Nicol F, Beckett GJ (1990) Hepatic iodothyronine 5′-deiodinase. The role of selenium. Biochem J 272: 537–540

Atkinson S, Kendall-Taylor P (1981) The stimulation of thyroid hormone secretion in vitro by thyroid-stimulating antibodies. J Clin Endocrinol Metab 53: 1263–1266

Barsano CP (1981) Environmental factors altering thyroid function and their assessment. Environ Health Perspect 38: 71–82

Basolo F, Pinchera A, Fugazzola L, Fontanini G, Elisei R, Romei C, Pacini F (1994) Expression of p21 ras protein as a prognostic factor in papillary thyroid cancer. Eur J Cancer 30A(2): 171–174

Bastomsky CH (1974) Effects of a chlorinated biphenyl mixture (Arochlor 1254) and DDT on biliary thyroxine excretion in rats. Endocrinology 95: 1150–1155

Bätge B, Dralle H, Padberg B, Herbay B, Schröder S (1992) Histology and immunocytochemistry of differentiated thyroid carcinomas do not predict radioiodine uptake: a clinicomorphological study of 62 recurrent or metastatic tumours. Virchows Arch [A] 421: 521–526

Baverstock K, Egloff B, Pinchera A, Ruchti C, Williams D (1992) Thyroid cancer after Chernobyl. Nature 359: 21–22

Beech SG, Walker SW, Dorrance AM, Arthur JR, Nicol F, Lee D, Beckett GJ (1993) The role of thyroidal type-I iodothyronine deiodinase in tri-iodothyronine production by human and sheep thyrocytes in primary culture. J Endocrinol 136: 361–370

Behne D, Hilmert H, Scheid S, Gessner H, Elger W (1988) Evidence for specific selenium target tissues and new biologically important selenoproteins. Biochim Biophys Acta 966: 12–21

Behne D, Kyriakopoulos A, Meinhold H, Köhrle J (1990) Identification of type I iodothyronine 5′-deiodinase as a selenoenzyme. Biochem Biophys Res Commun 173: 1143–1149

Beng CG, Wellby ML, Symons RG, Stuart S, Marshall J (1980) The effects of iopodate on the serum iodothyronine pattern in normal subjects. Acta Endocrinol (Copenh) 93: 175–178

Berlingieri MT, Santoro M, Battaglia C, Grieco M (1993) The adenovirus E1A gene blocks the differentiation of a thyroid epithelial cell line, however the neoplastic phenotype is achieved only after cooperation with other oncogenes. Oncogene 8: 249–255

Berry MJ, Banu L, Larsen PR (1991) Type I iodothyronine deiodinase is a selenocystein-containing enzyme. Nature 349: 438–440

Blondeau JP, Osty J, Francon J (1988) Characterization of the thyroid hormone transport system of isolated hepatocytes. J Biol Chem 263: 2685–2692

Bombick DW, Jankun J, Tullis K, Matsumara F (1988) 2,3,7,8-Tetrachlorodibenzo-*p*-dioxin causes increases in expression of c-erbA and levels of protein-tyrosine kinases in selected tissues of responsive mouse strains. Proc Natl Acad Sci USA 85: 4128–4132

Bongarzone I, Pierotti MA, Monzini N, Mondellini P, Manenti G, Doughi R, Pilotti S, Grieco M, Santoro M, Fusco A et al (1989) High frequency of activation of tyrosine kinase oncogenes in human papillary thyroid carcinoma. Oncogene 4: 1457–11462

Borek C, Guernsey DL, Ong A, Edelman IS (1983) Critical role played by thyroid hormone in induction of neoplastic transformation by chemical carcinogens in tissue culture. Proc Natl Acad Sci USA 80: 5749–4752

Borges M, Ingbar SH, Silva JE (1990) Iodothyronine deiodinase activities in FRTL-5 cells: predominance of type I 5′-deiodinase. Endocrinology 126: 3059–3068

Boye N, Laurberg P (1984) Deiodination of T4 to T3 and rT3 by microsomes from normal human thyroid tissue. Mol Cell Endocrinol 37: 295–299

Brabant G, Maenhaut C, Köhrle J, Scheumann G, Dralle H, Hoang-Vu C, Hesch RD, von zur Mühlen A, Vassart G, Dumont JE (1991) Human thyrotropin receptor gene: expression in thyroid tumors and correlation to markers of thyroid differentiation and dedifferentiation. Mol Cell Endocrinol 82: R7–R12

Brabant G, Bergmann P, Kirsch CM, Köhrle J, Hesch RD, von zur Mühlen A (1992) Early adaptation of thyrotropin and thyroglobulin secretion to experimentally decreased iodine supply in man. Metabolism 41: 1093–1096

Brabant G, Hoang-Vu C, Cetin C, Dralle H, Scheumann GFW, Moelne J, Hansson, Jansson S, Ericson LE, Nilsson M (1993) E-cadherin: a differentiation marker in thyroid malignancies. Cancer Res 53: 4987–4993

Buff K, Bründl A (1992) Specific binding of polychlorinated biphenyls to rat liver cytosol protein. Biochem Pharmacol 43: 965–970

Burk RF, Brown DG, Seely RJ, Scaief CC III (1972) Influence of dietary and injected selenium on whole-body retention, route of excretion, and tissue retention of 75(SeO3)2- in the rat. J Nutr 102: 1049–1056

Burmeister LA, Goumaz MO, Mariash CN, Oppenheimer JH (1992) Levothyroxine dose requirements for thyrotropin suppression in the treatment of differentiated thyroid cancer. J Clin Endocrinol Metab 75: 344–350

Byrne JJ, Carbone JP, Hanson EA (1987) Hypothyroidism and abnormalities in the kinetics of thyroid hormone metabolism in rats treated chronically with polychlorinated biphenyl and polybrominated biphenyl. Endocrinology 121: 520–527

Chanoine JP, Stein GS, Braverman LE, Shalhoub V, Lian JB, Huber CA, DeVito WJ (1992) Acidic fibroblast growth factor modulates gene expression in the rat thyroid in vivo. J Cell Biochem 50: 392–399
Chanoine JP, Braverman LE, Farwell AP, Safran M, Alex S, Dubord S, Leonard JL (1993) The thyroid gland is a major source of circulating T3 in the rat. J Clin Invest 91: 2709–2713
Chin WW, Carr FE, Burnside J, Darling DS (1993) Thyroid hormone regulation of thyrotropin gene expression. Recent Prog Horm Res 48: 393–414
Clark OH, Duh Q-Y (1990) Thyroid cancer. In: Greer MA (ed) The thyroid gland. Raven, New York, pp 537–571
Cody V (1985) Conformational analysis of environmental agents: use of X-ray crystallographic data to determine molecular reactivity. Environ Health Perspect 61: 163–183
Collins WT, Capen CC (1980) Ultrastructural and fuctional alterations of the rat thyroid gland produced by polychlorinated biphenyls compared with iodide excess and deficiency, and thyrotropin and thyroxine administration. Virchows Arch [B] 33: 213–231
Contempre B, Dumont JE, Bebe N, Thilly CH, Diplock AT, Vanderpas J (1991a) Effect of selenium supplementation in hypothyroid subjects of an iodine and selenium deficient area: the possible danger of indiscriminate supplementation of iodine-deficient subjects with selenium. J Clin Endocrinol Metab 73: 213–215
Contempre B, Vanderpas J, Dumont JE (1991b) Cretinism, thyroid hormones and selenium. Mol Cell Endocrinol 81: C193–C195
Costa A (1979) The use of X-ray contrast media in the treatment of hyperthyroidism. J Endocrinol Invest 2: 461–462
Curran PG, DeGroot LJ (1991) The effect of hepatic enzyme-inducing drugs on thyroid hormones and the thyroid gland. Endocr Rev 12: 135–150
DeGroot LJ (1993) Effects of irradiation on the thyroid gland. Endocrinol Metab Clin North Am 22(3): 607–615
DeGroot LJ, Nakai A, Sakurai A, Macchia E (1989) The molecular basis of thyroid hormone action. J Endocrinol Invest 12: 843–861
Demeure MJ, Hughes-Fulford M, Goretzki PE, Duh Q-Y, Clark OH (1990) Actin architecture of cultured human thyroid cancer cells: predictor of differentiation? Surgery 108: 986–993
Demeure MJ, Damsky CH, Elfman F, Goretzki PE, Wong MG, Clark OH (1992) Invasion by cultured human follicular thyroid cancer correlates with increased betal integrins and production of proteases. World J Surg 16: 770–776
Derwahl M, Hamacher C, Papageorgiu G, Zbaeren J, Schatz H, Studer H (1993) Expression of Gs protein alpha subunit in thyroid adenomas. Exp Clin Endocrinol 101: 51–53
Di Renzo MF, Narsimhan RP, Olivero M, Bretti S, Giordano S, Medico E, Gaglia P, Zara P, Comoglio PM (1991) Expression of the Met/HGF receptor in normal and neoplastic human tissues. Oncogene 6: 1997–2003
Di Renzo MF, Olivero M, Ferro S, Prat M, Bongarzone I, Pilotti S, Belfiore A, Costantino A, Vigneri R, Pierotti MA et al (1992) Overexpression of the c-MET/HGF receptor gene in human thyroid carcinomas. Oncogene 7: 2549–2553
Dockhorn-Dwonrniczak B, Schroeder S, Dantcheva R, Toetsch M, Stuecker A, Broemmelkamp E, Bankfalvi A, Boecker W, Schmid KW (1993) The role of p53 tumor suppressor gene in thyroid cancer. Exp Clin Endocrinol 101: 39–46
Dumont JE, Lamy F, Roger P, Maenhaut C (1992) Physiological and pathological regulation of thyroid cell proliferation and differentiation by thyrotropin and other factors. Physiol Rev 72: 667–697
Edmonds CJ, Tellez M (1988) Hyperthyroidism and thyroid cancer. Clin Endocrinol 28: 253–259
Eggo M, Sheppard MC (1994) Autocrine growth factors produced in the thyroid. Mol Cell Endocrinol 100: 97–102
Elisei R, Pinchera A, Romei C, Gryczynska M, Pohl V, Maenhaut C, Fugazzola L, Pacini F (1994) Expression of thyrotropin receptor (TSH-R), thyroglobulin, thyroperoxidase, and calcitonin messenger ribonucleic acids in thyroid carcinomas: evidence of TSH-R gene transcript in medullary histotype. J Clin Endocrinol Metab 78(4): 867–871
Erickson VJ, Cavalieri RR, Rosenberg LL (1982) Thyroxine-5′-deiodinase of rat thyroid, but not that of liver, is dependent on thyrotropin. Endocrinology 111: 434–440

Erkenbrack DE, Rosenberg LL (1986) Binding of thyroid hormones to nuclear extracts of thyroid cells. Endocrinology 119: 311–317

Ezaki H, Ebihara S, Fujimoto Y, Iida F, Ito K, Kuma K, Izuo M, Makiuchi M, Oyamada H, Matoba N, Yagawa K (1992) Analysis of thyroid carcinoma based on material registerd in Japan during 1977–1986 with special reference to predominance of papillary type. Cancer 70: 808–814

Farid NR, Shi Y, Zou M (1994) Molecular basis of thyroid cancer. Endocr Rev 15(2): 202–232

Farwell AP, Leonard JL (1992) Dissociation of actin polymerization and enzyme inactivation in the hormonal regulation of type II iodothyronine 5′-deiodinase activity in astrocytes. Endocrinology 131: 721–728

Farwell AP, DiBenedetto DJ, Leonard JL (1993) Thyroxine targets different pathways of internalization of type II iodothyronine 5′-deiodinase in astrocytes. J Biol Chem 268: 5055–5062

Franceschi S, Boyle P, Maisonneuve P, La Vecchia C, Burt AD, Kerr DJ, MacFarlane GJ (1993) The epidemiology of thyroid carcinoma. Crit Rev Oncog 4: 25–52

Francis Lang H, Zannini M, De Felice M, Berlingieri MT, Fusco A, Di Lauro R (1992) Multiple mechanisms of interference between transformation and differentiation in thyroid cells. Mol Cell Biol 12: 5793–5800

Gaitan E, Lindsay RH, Reichert RD, Ingbar SH, Cooksey RC, Legan J, Meydrech EF, Hill J, Kubota K (1989) Antithyroid and goitrogenic effects of millet: role of C-glycosylflavones. J Clin Endocrinol Metab 68: 707–714

Gärtner R (1993) Growth factors of the thyroid. Exp Clin Endocrinol 101: 83–91

Gärtner R, Bechtner G, Stuebner D, Greil W (1990) Growth regulation of porcine thyroid follicles in-vitro by growth factors. Horm Metab Res Suppl 23: 61–67

Goretzki P (1996) Establishment and characterization of three human thyrocyte cell lines from one patient presenting with p53 and G-protein (gsp) mutations. Cancer Res (submitted)

Goretzki PE, Frilling A, Simon D, Roeher H-D (1990) Growth regulation of normal thyroids and thyroid tumors in man. Recent Results Cancer Res 118: 48–63

Goretzki P, Gorelov V, Weissmann K, Dumon K, Ebeling B, Simon D, Gyenes M, Palm D, Mollner S, Pfeuffer T, Bosilij B, Lyons J, Roeher HD (1993) Mutation and expression of alpha Gs in differentiated thyroid carcinoma (DTC) and medullary thyroid carcinoma (MTC). Exp Clin Endocrinol 101: 54–59

Green WL (1991) Effect of drugs on thyroid hormone metabolism. In: Wu S-Y (ed) Thyroid hormone metabolism. Blackwell, Boston, pp 239–265

Greer M, Grimm Y, Studer H (1968) Qualitative changes in the secretion of thyroid hormones induced by iodine deficiency. Endocrinology 83: 1193–1198

Grieco M, Santoro M, Berlingieri MT, Donghi R, Pierotti MA, Della Porta G, Fusco A, Vecchio G (1988) Molecular cloning of PTC, a new oncogene found activated in human thyroid papillary carcinomas and their lymph node metastases. Ann N Y Acad Sci 551: 380–384

Grieco M, Santoro M, Berlingieri MT, Melillo RM, Donghi R, Bongarzone I, Pierotti MA, Della Porta G, Fusco A, Vecchio G (1990) PTC is a novel rearranged form of the ret proto-oncogene and is frequently detected in vivo in human thyroid papillary carcinomas. Cell 60: 557–563

Gross M, Oertel M, Müller Brechlin A, Rokos H, Körhrle J (1992) Cellular hierarchy of selenium incorporation into 5′deiodinase in LLC-PK1 cells (Abstr). Ann Endocrinol (Paris)

Gross M, Oertel M, Köhrle J (1995) Differential selenium-dependent regulation of type I 5′-deiodinase and glutathione peroxidase in the porcine epithelial kidney cell line LLC-PK1. Biochem J 306(3): 851–856

Hales IB, McElduff A, Crummer P, Clifton-Bligh P, Delbridge L, Hoschl R, Poole A, Reeve TS, Wilmshurst E, Wiseman J (1992) Does Graves' disease or thyrotoxicosis affect the prognosis of thyroid cancer. J Clin Endocrinol Metab 75: 886–889

Hashimoto T, Matsubara F, Mizukami Y, Miyazaki I, Michigishi T, Yanaihara N (1990) Tumor markers and oncogene expression in thyroid cancer using biochemical and immunohistological studies. Endocrinol Jpn 37: 247–254

Herrmann MA, Hay ID, Bartelt DH Jr, Ritland SR, Dahl RJ, Grant CS, Jenkins RB (1991) Cytogenetic and molecular genetic studies of follicular and papillary thyroid cancers. J Clin Invest 88: 1596–1604

Hesch RD (1981) The "low T3-syndrome". Academic, London

Hishinuma A, Kasai K, Ichimura K, Emoto T, Shimoda S (1992) Effects of epidermal growth factor, phorbol ester, and retinoic acid on hormone synthesis and morphology in porcine thyroid follicles cultured in collagen gel. Thyroid 2: 351–359

Hoang-Vu C, Dralle H, Scheumann G, Maenhaut C, Horn R, von zur Mühlen A, Brabant G (1992a) Gene expression of differentiation and dedifferentiation markers in normal and malignant human thyroid tissues. Exp Clin Endocrinol 100: 51–56

Hoang-Vu C, Dralle H, Schroeder S, Oertel M, Köhrle J, Hesch RD, von zur Mühlen A, Brabant G (1992b) The nude rat is established as a model for endocrine studies: regulation of thyroid function and xenotransplantation of a thyroid tumor cell line. Lab Anim Sci 42(2): 1–4

Hoang-Vu C, Cetin Y, Scheumann GFW, Behrends J, Horn R, von zur Mühlen A, Dralle H, Brabant G (1993) Expression of cellular adhesion molecule, E-cadherin, in normal human thyrocytes, and in differentiated and undifferentiated thyroid carcinomas. Exp Clin Endocrinol 101: 78–82

Hörmann R, Saller B, Mann K (1990) Evaluation of the ratio of T3 release stimulating antibodies to TSH-binding inhibiting antibodies during the course of Graves' disease. Horm Metab Res 22: 183–187

Ikeda T, Honda M, Murakami I, Kuno S, Mokuda O, Tokumori Y, Tominaga M, Mashiba H (1985) Effect of TSH on conversion of T4 to T3 in perfused rat kidney. Metabolism 34(11): 1057–1060

Ishii H, Inada M, Tanaka K, Mashio Y, Naito K, Nishikawa M, Imura H (1981) Triiodothyronine generation from thyroxine in human thyroid: enhanced conversion in Graves' thyroid tissue. J Clin Endocrinol Metab 52: 1211–1217

Ishii H, Inada M, Tanaka K, Mashio Y, Naito K, Nishikawa M, Matsuzuka F, Kuma K, Imura H (1982) Sequential deiodination of thyroxine in human thyroid gland. J Clin Endocrinol Metab 55: 890–896

Ishii H, Inada M, Tanaka K, Mashio Y, Naito K, Nishikawa M, Matsuzuka F, Kuma K, Imura H (1983) Induction of outer and inner ring monodeiodinases in human thyroid gland by thyrotropin. J Clin Endocrinol Metab 57: 500–505

Ito A, Watanabe H, Naito M, Aoyama H, Nakagawa Y, Fujimoto N (1986) Induction of thyroid tumors in (C57BL/6N X C3H/N)F1 mice by oral administration of 9-3′,4′,5′6′-tetrachloro-*o*-carboxyphenyl-6-hydroxy-2,4,5,7-tetraoido-3-isoxanthonesodium (Food Red 105, Rose Bengal B). JNCI 77: 277–281

Ito T, Seyama T, Iwamoto KS, Hayashi T, Mizuno T, Tsuyama N, Dohi K, Nakamura N, Akiyama M (1993) In vitro irradiation is able to cause RET oncogene rearrangement. Cancer Res 53: 2940–2943

Kamikubo K, Nayfeh SN, Chae C-B (1992) Differential regulation of multiple c-erbA expression by thyrotropin, insulin and insulin-like growth factor I in rat thyroid FRTL-5 cells. Mol Cell Endocrinol 84: 219–225

Kazakov VS, Demidchik EP, Astakova LN (1992) Thyroid cancer after Chernobyl. Nature 359: 21–22

Kimura H, Yamashita S, Namba H, Tominaga T, Tsuruta M, Yokoyama N, Izumi M, Nagataki S (1992a) Interleukin-1 inhibits thyroid carcionoma cell growth. J Clin Endocrinol Metab 75: 596–602

Kimura H, Yamashita S, Namba H, Usa T, Fujiyama K, Tsuruta M, Yokoyama N, Izumi M, Nagataki S (1992b) Impairment of the TSH signal transduction system in human thyroid carcinoma cells. Exp Cell Res 203: 402–406

Kinlaw WB, Schwartz HL, Oppenheimer JH (1985) Decreased serum triiodothyronine in starving rats is due primarily to diminished thyroidal secretion of thyroxine. J Clin Invest 75: 1238–1241

Kohn AD, Chan J, Grieco D, Nikodem VM, Aloj SM, Kohn LD (1989) Thyrotropin increases malic enzyme messenger ribonucleic acid levels in rat FRTL-5 thyroid cells. Mol Endocrinol 3: 532–538

Köhrle J (1983) Untersuchungen zur Charakterisierung der enzymatischen Dejodierung von L-Thyroxin und anderen Jodthyroninen durch Rattenlebermikrosomen - Befunde für die Existenz nur einer Jodthyronin-Dejodase. Published privately, Hannover

Köhrle J (1990) Thyrotropin (TSH) action on thyroid hormone deiodination and secretion: one aspect of thyrotropin regulation of thyroid cell biology. Horm Metab Res Suppl 23: 18–28

Köhrle J (1992) The trace components - selenium and flavonoids - affect iodothyronine deiodinases, thyroid hormone transport and TSH regulation. Acta Med Austriaca 19 Suppl 1: 13–17

Köhrle J (1994a) Thyroid hormone deiodination in target tissues – a regulatory role for the trace element selenium? Exp Clin Endocrinol 102: 63–89

Köhrle J (1994b) Von Pflanzenextrakten zu Hormonantagonisten - Neue experimentelle Konzepte zur Hyperthyreosetherapie. In: Reinwein D, Weinheimer B (eds) Schilddrüse 1993. de Gruyter, Berlin

Köhrle J (1995) Jod: Selen und Jodversorgung – endokrinologische Zusammenhänge. In: Kruse-Jarres JD (ed) VII Stuttgarter Mineralstoff-Symposium, 3-4 June 1994: Mineralstoffe, Spurenelemente, Vitamine: Risikofaktoren - Meßverfahren - Präventivmassnahmen. Biosymposia, Stuttgart

Köhrle J, Müller MJ, Ködding R, Seitz HJ, Hesch RD (1982) pH dependency of iodothyronine metabolism in isolated perfused rat liver. Biochem J 202: 669–675

Köhrle J, Fang SL, Yang Y, Irmscher K, Hesch RD, Pino S, Alex S, Braverman LE (1989) Rapid effects of the flavonoid EMD 21388 on serum thyroid hormone binding and thyrotropin regulation in the rat. Endocrinology 125: 532–537

Köhrle J, Hesch RD, Leonard JL (1991) Intracellular pathways of iodothyronine metabolism. In: Braverman LE, Utiger RD (eds) Werner and Ingbar's the thyroid - a fundamental and clinical text, 6th edn. Lippincott, Philadelphia, pp 144–189

Köhrle J, Oertel M, Hoang-Vu C, Schnieders F, Brabant G (1993) Type I 5′-deiodinase – a marker for differentiated thyroid carcinoma? Exp Clin Endocrinol 101 Suppl 3: 60–72

Köhrle J, Groß M, Fekete E, Goretzki P, Brabant G (1994) Differential expression of type I 5′-deiodinase and other selenoproteins in human thyroid carcinoma and various epithelial cell lines (Abstr). Eur J Endocrinol 130: 41

Kraiem Z, Sadeh O, Yosef M (1991) Iodide uptake and organification, tri-iodothyronine secretion, cyclic AMP accumulation and cell proliferation in an optimized system of human thyroid follicles cultured in collagen gel suspended in serum-free medium. J Endocrinol 131: 499–506

Krenning EP, Docter R (1991) Plasma membrane transport of thyroid hormone. In: Hennemann G (ed) Thyroid hormone metabolism. Dekker, New York, pp 107–131

Kubota K, Uchimura H, Mitsuhashi T, Chiu SC, Kuzuya N, Nagataki S (1984) Effects of intrathyroidal metabolism of thyroxine on thyroid hormone secretion: increased degradation of thyroxine in mouse thyroids stimulated chronically with thyrotropin. Acta Endocrinol (Copenh) 105: 57–65

Kumar MS, Chiang T, Deodhar SD (1979) Enhancing effect of thyroxine on tumor growth and metastases in syngeneic mouse tumor systems. Cancer Res 39: 3515–3518

Langsteger W, Koltringer P, Wolf G, Dominik K, Buchinger W, Binter G, Lax S, Eber O (1993) The impact of geographical, clinical, dietary and radiation-induced features in epidemiology of thyroid cancer. Eur J Cancer 29A(11): 1547–1553

Laurberg P (1978) Selective inhibition of TSH secretion of triiodothyronines from the perfused canine thyroid by propylthiouracil. Endocrinology 103: 900–905

Laurberg P (1980) Iodothyronine release from the perfused canine thyroid. Acta Endocrinol (Copenh) Suppl 236

Laurberg P (1981) Iodothyronine secretion from perfused dog thyroid lobes after prolonged thyrotropin treatment in vivo. Endocrinology 109: 1560–1565

Laurberg P (1982) The effect of some iodine-containing radiocontrast agents on iodothyronine secretion from the perfused canine thyroid. Endocrinology 111: 1904–1908

Lazzaro D, Price M, De Felice M, Di Lauro R (1991) The transcription factor TTF-1 is expressed at the onset of thyroid and lung morphogenesis and in restricted regions of the foetal brain. Development 113: 1093–1104

Lemoine NR, Mayall ES, Wyllie FS, Farr CJ, Hughes D, Padua RA, Thurston V, Williams ED, Wynford-Thomas D (1988) Activated *ras* oncogenes in human thyroid cancers. Cancer Res 48: 4459–4463
Leonard JL, (1991) Identification and structure analysis of iodothyronine deiodinases. In: Greer MA (ed) The thyroid gland. Raven, New York, pp 285–321
Leonard JL, Rennke H, Kaplan MM, Larsen PR (1982) Subcellular distribution of iodothyronine 5′-deiodinase in cerebral cortex from hypothyroid rats. Biochim Biophys Acta 718: 109–119
Leonard JL, Ekenbarger DM, Frank SJ, Farwell AP, Köhrle J (1991) Localization of type I iodothyronine 5′deiodinase to the basolateral plasma membrane of rat kidney and LLC-PK1 renal cortical cells. J Biol Chem 266: 11262–11269
Leuthauser SWC, Guernsey DL (1987) Thyroid hormone affects the expression of neoplastic transformation induced by DNA-transfection. Cancer Lett 35: 321–326
Lopez CA, Hsiao W-LW, Weinstein IB (1989) Effects of triiodothyronine and tamoxifen on cell transformation induced by an activated c-Ha-*ras* oncogene. Cancer Res 49: 895–898
Mashita K, Kawamura S, Kishino B, Kimura H, Nonaka K, Tarui S (1982) Effects of iodide and propylthiouracil on the release of 3,5,3′-triiodothyronine and of cyclic adenosine 3′,5′-monophosphate from perfused rat thyroids. Endocrinology 110(3): 1023–1029
Matsuo K, Tang S-H, Fagin JA (1991) Allelotype of human thyroid tumors: loss of chromosome 11q13 sequences in follicular neoplasms. Mol Endocrinol 5: 1873–1879
Matsuo K, Friedman E, Gejman PV, Fagin JA (1993a) The thyrotropin receptor (TSH-R) is not an oncogene for thyroid tumors: structural studies of the TSH-R and the alpha-subunit of Gs in human thyroid neoplasms. J Clin Endocrinol Metab 76: 1446–1451
Matsuo K, Tang S-H Zeki K, Gutman RA, Fagin JA (1993b) Aberrant deoxyribonucleic acid methylation in human thyroid tumors. J Clin Endocrinol Metab 77(4): 991–995
Mazzaferri EL (1990) Thyroid cancer and Graves' disease. J Clin Endocrinol Metab 70: 826–829
McKinney JD (1985) The molecular basis of chemical toxicity. Environ Health Perspect 61: 5–10
McKinney JD, Chae K, Oatley SJ, Blake CCF (1985) Molecular interactions of toxic chlorinated dibenzo-*p*-dioxins and dibenzofurans with thyroxine binding prealbumin. J Med Chem 28: 375–381
Medeiros-Neto G, Targovnik HM, Vassart G (1993) Defective thyroglobulin synthesis and secretion causing goiter and hypothyroidism. Endocr Rev 14: 165–183
Meinhold H, Campos-Barros A, Walzog B, Köhler R, Müller F, Behne D (1993) Effects of selenium and iodine deficiency on type I, type II, and type III iodothyronine deiodinases and circulating hormone levels in the rat. Exp Clin Endocrinol 100: 87–93
Miyamoto M, Sugawa H, Mori T, Hase K, Kuma K, Imura H (1988) Epidermal growth factor receptors on cultured neoplastic human thyroid cells and effects of epidermal growth factor and thyroid-stimulating hormone on their growth. Cancer Res 48: 3652–3656
Mooradian AD, Schwartz HL, Mariash CN, Oppenheimer JH (1985) Transcellular and transnuclear transport of 3,5,3′-triiodothyronine in isolated hepatocytes. Endocrinology 117: 2449–2456
Müller MJ, Köhrle J, Hesch RD, Seitz HJ (1982) Effect of cycloAMP on iodothyronine metabolism in the isolated perfused rat liver. Biochem Int 5: 495–501
Mulligan LM, Kwok JB, Healey CS, Elsdon MJ, Eng C, Gardner E, Love DR, Mole SE, Moore JK, Papi L et al (1993) Germ-line mutations of the RET proto-oncogene in multiple endocrine neoplasia type 2A. Nature 363: 458–460
Nakamura H, Imura H (1988) Existence of nuclear thyroid hormone receptors in the porcine thyroid gland and the rat thyroid cell line FRTL-5. Acta Endocrinol (Copenh) 117: 116–124
Namba H, Gutman RA, Matsuo K, Alvarez A, Fagin JA (1990a) H-*ras* protooncogene mutations in human thyroid neoplasms. J Clin Endocrinol Metab 71: 223–229
Namba H, Rubin SA, Fagin JA (1990b) Point mutations of *ras* oncogenes are an early event in thyroid tumorigenesis. Mol Endo crinol 4: 1474–1479
Namba H, Yamashita S, Morita S, Villadolid MC, Kimura H, Yokoyama N, Izumi M, Ishikawa N, Ito K, Nagataki S (1993) Retinoic acid inhibits human thyroid peroxidase and thyroglobulin gene expression in cultured human thyrocytes. J Endocrinol Invest 16: 87–93
Naumann A, Naumann J, Witeska A, Dutkiewicz M (1993) 5′-Deiodinase type I in human kidney cancer (Abstr). J Endocrinol Invest 16 Suppl 2: 76

Nishida M, Kumamoto T, Yano S, Yamaguchi T, Otsuka M, Kawada J (1991) Unusually high levels of thyroid hormones in isolated and/or monolayer-cultured pig thyroid epithelial cells. Naturwissenschaften 78: 509–511

O'Sullivan C, Barton CM, Staddon SL, Brown CL, Lemoine NR (1991) Activating point mutations of the *gsp* oncogene in hunman thyroid adenomas. Mol Carcinog 4: 345–349

Oertel M, Hesch RD, Köhrle J (1991) Type I 5'deiodinase and its 27 kDa substrate binding subunit are expressed in FRTL-5 but not in human FTC-133 follicular thyroid carcinoma cells. In: Gordon A, Gross J, Hennemann G (eds) Progress in thyroid research, Baalkema, Rotterdam, pp 685–688

Oertel M, Gross M, Rokos H, Köhrle J (1993) Selenium-dependent regulation of type I 5'-deiodinase expression. Am J Clin Nutr 57: 313S–314S

Oppenheimer JH, Schwartz HL, Mariash CN, Kinlaw WB, Wong NCW, Freake HC (1987) Advances in our understanding of thyroid hormone action at the cellular level. Endocr Rev 8: 288–308

Ottevanger PB, Hermus A, Smals AGH, Kloppenborg PWC (1992) TSH-dependent production of T4 and t3 by metastases of thyroid carcinoma. Acta Endocrinol (Copenh) 127: 413–415

Parma J, Duprez L, Van Sande J, Cochaux P, Gervy C, Mockel J, Dumont J, Vassart G (1993) Somatic mutations in the thyrotropin receptor gene cause hyperfunctioning thyroid adenomas (see comments). Nature 365: 649–651

Paul SJ, Sisson JC (1990) Thyrotoxicosis caused by thyroid cancer. Endocrinol Metab Clin North Am 19(3): 593–612

Peeters R, Buys N, Vanmontfort D, Van Isterdael J, Decuypere E, Kühn ER (1992) Preferential release of tri-iodothyronine following stimulation by thyrotrophin or thyrotrophin-releasing hormone in sheep of different ages. J Endocrinol 132: 93–100

Pesatori AC, Consonni D, Tironi A, Zocchetti C, Fini A, Bertazzi PA (1993) Cancer in a young population in a dioxin-contaminated area. Int J Epidemiol 22(6): 1010–1013

Pilo A, Iervasi G, Vitek F, Ferdeghini M, Cazzuola F, Bianchi R (1990) Thyroidal and peripheral production of 3,5,3'-triiodothyronine in humans by multicompartmental analysis. Am J Physiol 258: E715–E726

Pisarev MA, Juvenal GJ, Kleiman de Pisarev DL, Chazenbalk GD, Krawiec L, Valsecchi RM(1986) Subcellular location and binding of [^{125}I]-triiodothyronine in calf thyroid. Horm Metab Res 18: 318–322

Pontecorvi A, Robbins J (1989) The plasma membrane and thyroid hormone entry into cells. Trends Endocrinol Metab 1: 90–94

Rao GS, Rao ML, Thilmann A, Quednau HD (1981) Study of fluxes at low concentrations of L-tri-iodothyronine with rat liver cells and their plasma-membrane vesicles. Biochem J 198: 457–466

Refetoff S, Weiss RE, Usala SJ (1993) The syndromes of resistance to thyroid hormone. Endocr Rev 14: 348–399

Reinwein D, Benker G, Windeck R, Eigler FW, Leder L-D, Mlynek M-L, Creutzig H, Reiners C (1989) Erstsymptome bei Schilddrüsenmalignomen: Einfluß von Alter und Geschlecht in einem Jodmangelgebiet. Dtsch Med Wochenschr 114: 775–782

Rochefort P, Feunteun J, Desmoulins C (1993) Papillary thyroid carcinomas, thyroid dysgenesis, and thyroid hypertrophy in transgenic mice expressing a human activated *ras* gene driven by a thyroglobulin promoter. J Endocrinol Invest 16 Suppl 2: 2

Roger PP, Rickaert F, Lamy F, Authelet M, Dumont JE (1989) Actin stress fiber disruption and tropomyosin isoform switching in normal thyroid epithelial cells stimulated by thyrotropin and phorbol esters. Exp Cell Res 182: 1–13

Ron E, Lubin J, Schneider AB (1992) Thyroid cancer incidence. Nature 360: 113

Ron E, Preston DL, Mabuchi K, Thompson DE, Soda M (1994) Cancer incidence in atomic bomb survivors. IV. Comparison of cancer incidence and mortality. Radiat Res 137 2 Suppl: S98–S112

Safran M, Farwell AP, Leonard JL (1991) Evidence that type II 5'-deiodinase is not a selenoprotein. J Biol Chem 266: 13477–13480

Safran M, Farwell AP, Rokos H, Leonard JL (1993) Structural requirements of iodothyronines for the rapid inactivation and internalization of type II iodothyronine 5'-deiodinase in glial cells. J Biol Chem 268: 14224–14229

Sakurai A, Nakai A, DeGroot LJ (1989) Expression of three forms of thyroid hormone receptor in human tissues. Mol Endocrinol 3: 392–399

Santoro M (1990) The ret proto-oncogene is consistently expressed in human pheochromocytoma and thyroid medullary carcinoma. Oncogene 5: 1595–1598

Santoro M, Melillo RM, Grieco M, Berlingieri MT, Vecchio G, Fusco A (1993) The TRK and RET tyrosine kinase oncogenes cooperate with *ras* in the neoplastic transformation of a rat thyroid epithelial cell line. Cell Growth Diff 4: 77–84

Sarda AK, Singh MK, Bal S, Kapur A, Kapur M (1989) A report of four cases of thyroid cancer occurring in thyrotoxicosis and review of the literature. Jpn J Surg 19(3): 363–366

Schelfhout LJDM, van Muijen GNP, Fleuren GJ (1989) Expression of keratin 19 distinguishes papillary thyroid carcinoma from follicular carcinoma and follicular thyroid adenoma. Am J Clin Pathol 92: 654–658

Schmid KW (1993) Immunohistochemistry and in situ hybridisation in thyroid cancer. Exp Clin Endocrinol 101: 17–22

Schneider AB, Ron E, Lubin J, Stovall M, Gierlowski TC (1993) Dose-response relationships for radiation-induced thyroid cancer and thyroid nodules: evidence for the prolonged effects of radiation on the thyroid. J Clin Endocrinol Metab 77: 362–369

Schreck R, Schnieders F, Schmutzler C, Köhrle J (1994) Retinoids stimulate type I iodothyronine 5′-deiodinase activity in human follicular thyroid carcinoma cell lines. J Clin Endocrinol Metab 79(3): 791–798

Schröder-van der Elst J, Van der Heide D, Köhrle J (1991) In vivo effects of flavonoid EMD 21388 on thyroid hormone secretion and metabolism in the rat. Am J Physiol 261: E227–E232

Sellitti DF, Tseng Y-CL, Latham KR (1981) Effect of 3,5,3′-triiodo-l-thyronine on the incidence and growth kinetics of spontaneous mammary tumors in C3H/HeN mice. Cancer Res 41: 5015–5019

Selmi-Ruby S, Rousset B (1994) Thyroid hormone receptors in thyroid cells: expression and functional analysis. Eur J Endocrinol 130 Suppl 2: 49

Sharp B, Reed AW, Tamagna EI, Geffner DL, Hershman JM (1981) Treatment of hyperthyroidism with sodium ipodate (Oragrafin) in addition to propylthiouracil and propanolol. J Clin Endocrinol Metab 53: 622–625

Shi Y, Zou M, Farid NR (1993) Expression of thyrotrophin receptor gene in thyroid carcinoma is associated with good prognosis. Clin Endocrinol (Oxf) 39: 269–274

Short J, Ove P (1983) Synthesis of an hypothesis advocating a prominent role for the thyroid hormones in mammalian liver cell proliferation in vivo. Cytobios 38: 39–49

Siegel E (1976) Thyroxine and triiodothyronine influence cultured thyroid cells: alterations of morphology and mucosubstances (39314). Proc Soc Exp Biol Med 152: 1–5

Simon D, Goretzki PE, Gorelov V, Ebeling B, Roehrer HD (1993) Temperature gradient gel electrophoresis – a tool for screening of p53 mutations. Exp Clin Endocrinol 101: 47–50

Spanka M, Hesch R-D, Irmscher K, Köhrle J (1990) 5′-Deiodination in rat hepatocytes: effects of specific flavonoid inhibitors. Endocrinology 126: 1660–1667

Suarez HG, du Villard JA, Caillou B, Schlumberger M, Tubiana M, Parmentier C, Monier R (1988) Detection of activated *ras* oncogenes in human thyroid carcinomas. Oncogene 2: 403–406

Suarez HG, du Villard JA, Severino M, Caillou B, Schlumberger M, Tubiana M, Parmentier C, Monier R (1990) Presence of mutations of all three *ras* genes in human thyroid tumors. Oncogene 5: 565–570

Suarez HG, du Villard JA, Caillou B, Schlumberger M, Parmentier C (1991) Gsp mutations in human thyroid tumors. Oncogene 6: 677–679

Sugawara M, Lau R, Wasser HL, Nelson AM, Kuma K, Hershman JM (1984) Thyroid T4 5′-deiodinase activity in normal and abnormal human thyroid glands. Metabolism 33: 332–336

Sung LC, Cavalieri RR (1973) T3 Thyrotoxicosis due to metastatic thyroid carcinoma. J Clin Endocrinol Metab 36: 215–217

Takeichi M (1993) Cadherins in cancer: implications for invasion and metastasis. Curr Opin Cell Biol 5: 806–811

Toyoda N, Nishikawa M, Horimoto M, Yoshikawa N, Mori Y, Yoshimura M, Masaki H, Tanaka K, Inada M (1990) Graves' immunoglobulin G stimulates iodothyronine 5′-deiodinating activity in FRTL-5 rat thyroid cells. J Clin Endocrinol Metab 70: 1506–1511

Toyoda N, Nishikawa M, Mori Y, Gondou A, Ogawa Y, Yonemoto T, Yoshimura M, Masaki H, Inada M (1992a) Thyrotropin and triiodothyronine regulate iodothyronine 5′-deiodinase messenger ribonucleic acid levels in FRTL-5 rat thyroid cells. Endocrinology 131: 389–394

Toyoda N, Nishikawa M, Mori Y, Yoshimura M, Masaki H, Gondou A, Yonemoto T, Inada M (1992b) Identification of a 27-kilodalton protein with the properties of type I iodothyronine 5′-deiodinase in human thyroid gland. J Clin Endocrinol Metab 74: 533–538

Van Herle AJ, Agatep ML, Padua DN III, Totanes TL, Canlapan DV, Van Herle HML, Juillard GJF (1990) Effects of 13 *cis*-retinoic acid on growth and differentiation of human follicular carcinoma cells (UCLA RO 82 W-1) in vitro. J Clin Endocrinol Metab 71: 755–763

Vassart G, Dumont JE (1992) The thyrotropin receptor and the regulation of thyrocyte function and growth. Endocr Rev 3: 596–611

Vranckx R, Rouaze M, Savu L, Nunez EA, Beaumont C, Flink IL (1990) The hepatic biosynthesis of rat thyroxine binding globulin (TBG): demonstration, ontogenesis, and up-regulation in experimental hypothyroidism. Biochem Biophys Res Commun 167: 317–322

Wartofsky L, Burman KD (1993) Alterations in thyroid function in patients with systemic illness: the "euthyroid sick syndrome". Endocr Rev 3: 164–217

Weetman AP, Bennett GL, Wong WLT (1992) Thyroid follicular cells produce interleukin-8. J Clin Endocrinol Metab 75: 328–330

Westgren U, Melander A, Ingemansson S, Burger A, Tibblin S, Wahlin E (1977) Secretion of thyroxine, 3,5,3′-triiodothyronine and 3,3′,5′-triiodothyronine in euthyroid man. Acta Endocrinol (Copenh) 84: 281–289

Williams ED (1993) Radiation-induced thyroid cancer. Histopathology 23(4): 387–389

Wright PA, Lemoine NR, Mayall ES, Wyllie FS, Hughes D, Williams ED, Wynford-Thomas D (1989) Papillary and follicular thyroid carcinomas show a different pattern of *ras* oncogene mutation. Br J Cancer 60: 576–577

Wu S (1990) The effect of fasting on thyroidal T_4-5'monodeiodinating activity in mice. Acta Endocrinol (Copenh) 122: 175–180

Wu S-Y (1983) Thyrotropin-mediated induction of thyroidal iodothyronine monodeiodinases in the dog. Endocrinology 112: 417–424

Wu S-Y, Chopra IJ, Solomon DH, Johnson DE (1978) The effect of repeated administration of ipodate (Orographin) in hyperthyroidism. J Clim Endocrinol Metab 47: 1358–1362

Wu S-Y, Reggio R, Florsheim WH (1985) Characterization of thyrotropin-induced increase in iodothyronine monodeiodinating activity in mice. Endocrinology 116: 901–908

Wu S-Y, Reggio R, Florsheim W, Chopra IJ, Solomon DH (1987) Stimulation of thyroidal iodothyronine 5′-monodeiodinase by long-acting thyroid stimulator (LATS). Acta Endocrinol (Copenh) 114: 193–200

Wyllie FS, Lemoine NR, Williams ED, Wynford-Thomas D (1989) Structure and expression of nuclear oncogenes in multi-stage thyroid tumorigenesis. Br J Cancer 60: 561–565

Wynford-Thomas D (1993) Molecular basis of epithelial tumorigenesis: the thyroid model. Crit Rev Oncog 4: 1–23

Yen PM, Chin WW (1994) New advances in understanding the molecular mechanisms of thyroid hormone action. Trends Endocrinol Metab 5: 65–72

Young RA, Braverman LE, Rajatanavin R (1982) Low protein-high carbohydrate diet induces alterations in the serum thyronine-binding proteins in the rat. Endocrinology 110: 1607–1612

Zeki K, Nakano Y, Inokuchi N, Watanabe K, Morimoto I, Yamashita U, Eto S (1993) Autocrine stimulation of interleukin-1 in the growth of human thyroid carcinoma cell line NIM 1. J Clin Endocrinol Metab 76: 127–133

Zou M, Shi Y, Farid NR (1993) p53 mutations in all stages of thyroid carcinomas. J Clin Endocrinol Metab 77: 1054–1058

Transcytosis of IgG from the Basolateral to the Apical Membrane of Human Thyrocytes in Autoimmune Thyroid Disease

K.P. Zimmer, K.W. Schmid, W. Böcker, G.F.W. Scheumann, H. Dralle, J. Brämswig, and E. Harms

1 Introduction

The thyroid is affected by one of the most common organ-specific autoimmune diseases in humans. Three major autoantigens are involved in thyroid autoimmune disease: thyroglobulin (TG), thyroid peroxidase (TPO), and thyroid-stimulating hormone (TSH) receptor. Both hyperthyroidism and the development of goitre in Graves' disease are caused by stimulating autoantibodies against TSH receptors. Autoantibodies against TG and TPO can be detected in Graves' disease and Hashimoto's thyroiditis.

The thyroid gland offers many advantages for studying the pathogenesis of autoimmune diseases. The autoantigens which are involved in thyroid autoimmune disease have already been well characterised. The molecular structures of human TG, TPO and the human TSH receptor have been determined (Malthiery and Lissitzky 1987; Kimura et al. 1987; Libert et al. 1987, 1989; Nagayama et al. 1989). The biological functions of these three autoantigens are known (reviewed by Nunez and Pommier 1982; Taurog 1986; Nagayama and Rapoport 1992). Some of the functional properties of the thyroid autoantibodies have been discovered, but the pathogenetic role of autoantibodies against TG in autoimmune thyroiditis still remains to be determined (Henry et al. 1992; Schulz et al. 1992). Antibodies against TPO are found in the majority of patients suffering from Hashimoto's thyroiditis or Graves' disease (Strakvosch et al. 1982; Banga et al. 1991). In vitro assays have shown that they mediate cytotoxicity by complement (Khoury et al. 1981) and antibodies (Bogner et al. 1984). There are contradictory reports about their ability to inhibit the enzyme activity of TPO (Okamoto et al. 1989; Kohno et al. 1991; Saller et al. 1991). Antibodies against the TSH receptor

Current Topics in Pathology
Volume 91, K.W. Schmid/W. Böcker (Eds.)

are shown to activate or block the TSH receptors of follicular cells (ZAKARIJA and MCKENZIE 1987). Finally, the autoantibody repertoire and the autoantigenic domains involved in autoimmune thyroid disease have recently been defined on a molecular level (DAVIES et al. 1991; CHAZENBALK et al. 1993).

The immune response in autoimmune disease is considered to be initiated by antigen presentation similar to that occurring in infectious disease (reviewed by BRACIALE and BRACIALE 1991). It has been shown in antigen-presenting cells that autoantigens and HLA class II molecules associate in the lysosomal compartment and are transported to the cell surface, where they bind to the antigen receptors of $CD4^+$ lymphocytes. This activation of lymphocytes is responsible for the production of autoantibodies, the secretion of cytokines and the cytotoxic and suppressor action of $CD8^+$ lymphocytes.

Although our knowledge of the pathogenesis of thyroid autoimmune disease has improved over the past few years (PINCHERA et al. 1989; UTIGER 1991), few studies exist on the biological processes within the thyrocytes involved in thyroid autoimmune disease. For instance, the mechanism by which TPO presents to the immune system, which must occur for the formation of autoantibodies against TPO, has not yet been revealed. Neither is it known how TPO - the surface expression of which is restricted to the apical membrane of thyrocytes - is able to contact immunocompetent cells. The cellular pathway of autoantibodies gaining access to TPO on the apical membrane of thyrocytes is also obscure. Some studies have shown a lack of IgG on the apical membrane in thyrocytes of patients with thyroid autoimmune disease (WERNER et al. 1972; KALDERON and BOGAARS 1977; FUJIWARA et al. 1981; OKAMOTO et al. 1991), whereas others demonstrated the presence of IgG by direct immunofluorescence on this site (KOFFLER and FRIEDMAN 1964; KHOURY et al. 1984).

To our knowledge, the ultrastructural location of IgG in thyroid glands of patients with thyroid autoimmune disease has not been determined immunocytochemically. In the present study, we investigated the subcellular distribution of IgG in thyroid tissue of patients suffering from thyroid autoimmune disease, with special emphasis on IgG binding sites within thyrocytes. Using the immunogold technique and thawed thin frozen sections of thyroid tissue from patients with autoimmune thyroiditis, we gained evidence that IgG is transcytosed from the basolateral to the apical membrane of thyrocytes, thus being located close to the luminal face of the apical membrane. We propose a model concerning the intracellular translocation of proteins involved in thyroid autoimmune disease.

2 Material and Methods

2.1 Tissue Studied

Human thyroid glands from five patients with Graves' disease were obtained during surgery. The diagnosis was established on the basis of thyroid autoantibodies, histological examination and thyroid hormone levels. Small pieces (diameter

<2 mm) of thyroid tissue were fixed in 5% paraformaldehyde in 0.1 *M* PIPES over night at 4°C. Human fibroblasts were released from the culture dish by proteinase K treatment at 4°C followed by PMSF (phenylmethylsulphonyl fluoride) and pellets were fixed in the same way as described above.

2.2 Antibodies

A mouse monoclonal antibody against human IgG (Dako Diagnostika Hamburg, dilution 1:30), a biotinylated rabbit $F(ab')_2$ fragment against the Fc_γ fragment of human IgG (Dianova Hamburg, dilution 1:20) and a rabbit polyclonal antibody against TG (Dako Diagnostika, dilution of 1:150) were used. Goat $F(ab')_2$ fragment against human IgG, IgA and IgM (Dianova, dilution 1:10) were applied in control experiments. The binding sites of the primary antibodies were detected by gold-conjugated goat anti-mouse serum (6 and 12 nm diameter, Dianova, both diluted 1:10), streptavidin gold (5 and 10 nm diameter, Amersham Braunschweig, both diluted 1:40) and protein A-gold (prepared by the method of Slot and Geuze 1985).

2.3 Embedding of IgG and IgA in Gelatine

IgG (Sigma Deisenhofen) and IgA (Sigma) were mixed with 10% gelatine in PBS at a concentration of 10 mg/ml. After 50 μl of these solutions stiffened at 4°C, the droplets were fixed in 5% paraformaldehyde in 0.1 *M* PIPES for 1 h at room temperature. Subsequently they were cut into small pieces which were processed for cryoultramicrotomy.

2.4 Immunocytochemistry

The thyroid glands, fibroblasts and the pieces of IgG- and IgA-gelatine were prepared for sectioning and labelling of ultrathin frozen sections using the technique of Tokuyasu (Griffiths 1993), as previously described (Copeland et al. 1988; Zimmer et al. 1992). Sections were prepared by a Sorvall cryoultramicrotome MT 6000 at −100°C to −110°C. Immunolabelling was carried out at room temperature for 30–45 min for each antibody. The sections were viewed using a Philips 401 electron microscope.

2.5 Quantitation of Labelling

The number of gold particles per square micrometre was determined by point counting (Griffiths 1993). We determined the labelling density of IgG over the nuclei of thyrocytes and follicle lumina in three patients as well as on ultrathin sections of the IgG- or IgA-containing gelatine.

3 Results

In thyroid tissue of patients suffering from autoimmune thyroiditis, IgG molecules were immunolocalised in the intercellular space, associated with bundles of collagen, vessels and erythrocytes. They were found on the basolateral membrane of thyrocytes. Additionally, a high number of IgG molecules were seen in follicular lumina, most of them being situated close to the apical membrane (Fig. 1). Within thyrocytes IgG was located in transport vesicles (Fig. 2) and transcytotic vacuoles (Fig. 3). This labelling pattern was obtained using both the biotinylated $F(ab')_2$ fragments against the human γ chain visualised by streptavidin gold and a mouse monoclonal antibody against human IgG visualised by gold-conjugated goat anti-mouse immunoglobulins. The number of gold particles found within follicular lumina ranged from 12.8 to 0.3 gold particles/μm^2.

To ensure the specificity of IgG labelling, several control experiments were performed. A negligible background was obtained after preincubation of sections

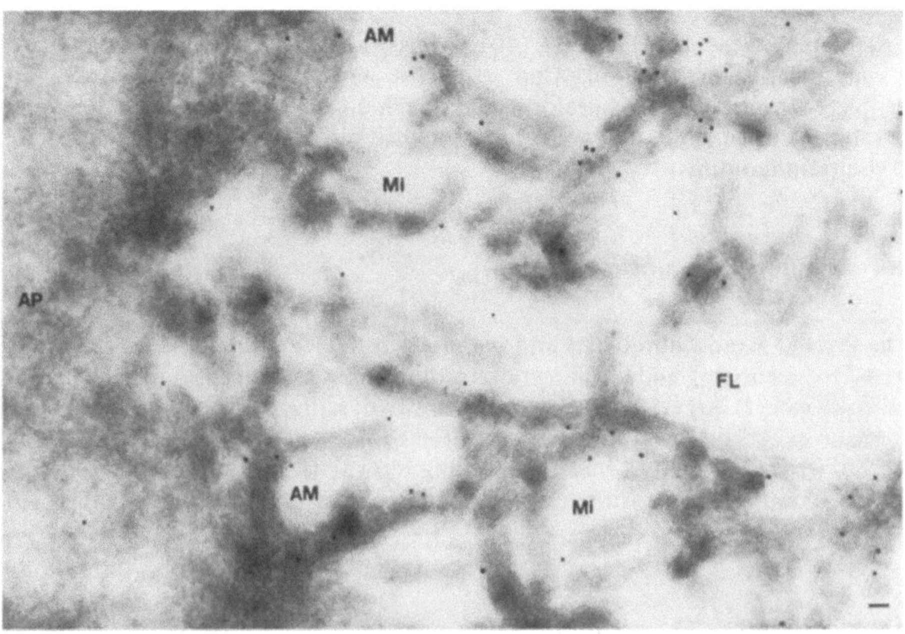

Fig. 1. Thin frozen section of a thyrocyte obtained from patient 1 is labelled by the monoclonal antibody against human IgG and gold-conjugated goat anti-mouse IgG. Numerous gold particles are present adjacent to the microvillus (*Mi*) membrane of the follicular lumen (*FL*). *AP*, apical pole; *AM*, apical membrane. *Bar*, 0.5 μm

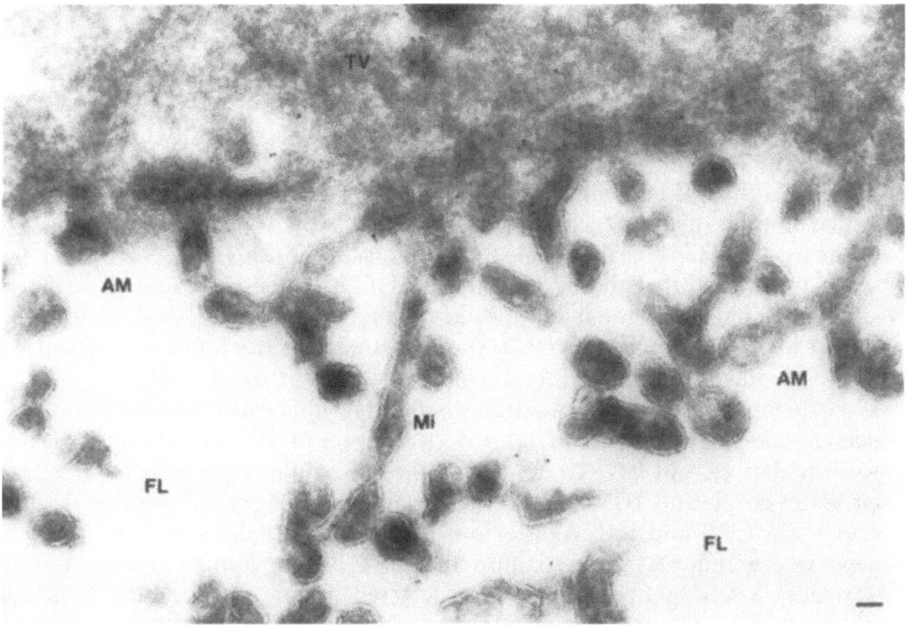

Fig. 2. Thin frozen section of a thyrocyte labelled by the biotinylated rabbit $F(ab')_2$ fragments against the Fc_γ fragment of human IgG and streptavidin gold 5 nm shows IgG at the apical membrane (*AM*) in addition to a transport vesicle (*TV*) filled with IgG. *Mi*, Microvilli; *FL*, follicular lumen. *Bar*, 0.5 μm

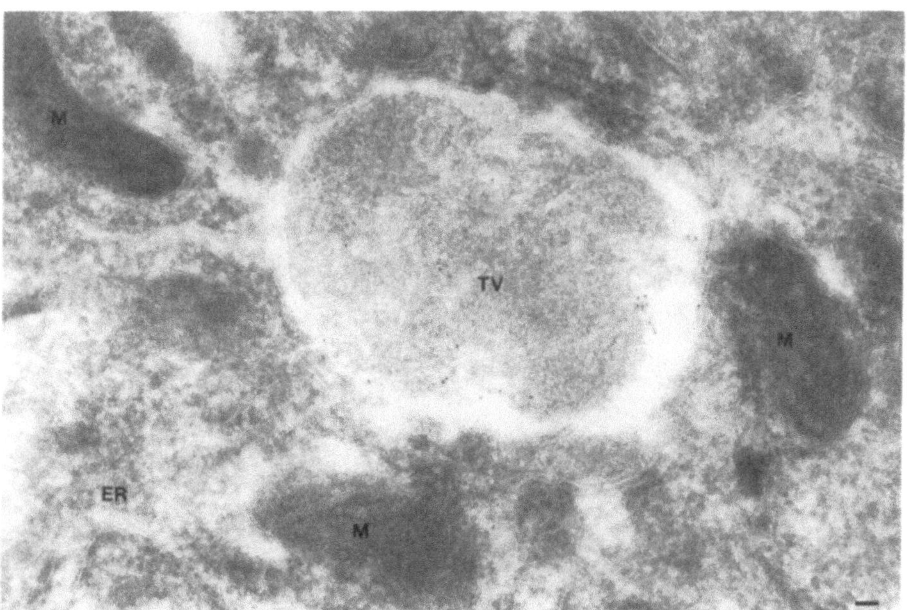

Fig. 3. Thin frozen section of a thyrocyte labelled as described in Fig. 2. A large membrane-bound organelle contains IgG, possibly a transcytotic vacuole (*TV*). *M*, mitochondria; *ER*, endoplasmic reticulum. *Bar*, 0.5 μm

with $F(ab')_2$ fragments against human IgG prior to the labelling procedure. No IgG could be detected in sections of cultured fibroblasts with any antibody tested (Fig. 4). To demonstrate the specificity of IgG within follicular lumina, the labelling density in the follicular lumen was compared to that of the nucleus. Quantitative evaluation of the IgG labelling (Fig. 5) revealed that the average labelling over the follicular lumina (83.6–167.5 μm^2 evaluated) was 5.3–12.8 times higher than that over the nuclei (43.0–66.5 μm^2 evaluated). The last is considered to be unspecific. These values reveal that the background of the IgG labelling is negligible. Since labelling with the monoclonal antibody against IgG was almost similar to labelling obtained by the biotinylated $F(ab')_2$ fragments against the human γ chain (not shown), streptavidin gold binding to endogenous biotin was excluded.

We further addressed the question whether IgG molecules are present in areas which contain high amounts of TG. Co-localisation of TG and IgG may suggest autoantibodies against TG. To determine the subcellular sites with putative co-localisation of IgG and TG, we performed double labelling experiments with antibodies against TG and IgG. As previously shown, the highest amount of TG is present in the endoplasmic reticulum and the follicular lumina (ZIMMER et al. 1992). Only a few IgG molecules were detected in the centre of the follicular lumina, where TG is present at a high concentration. As shown in single labelling experiments, the majority of IgG molecules in the follicle lumina are situated close to the apical membrane (Fig. 6).

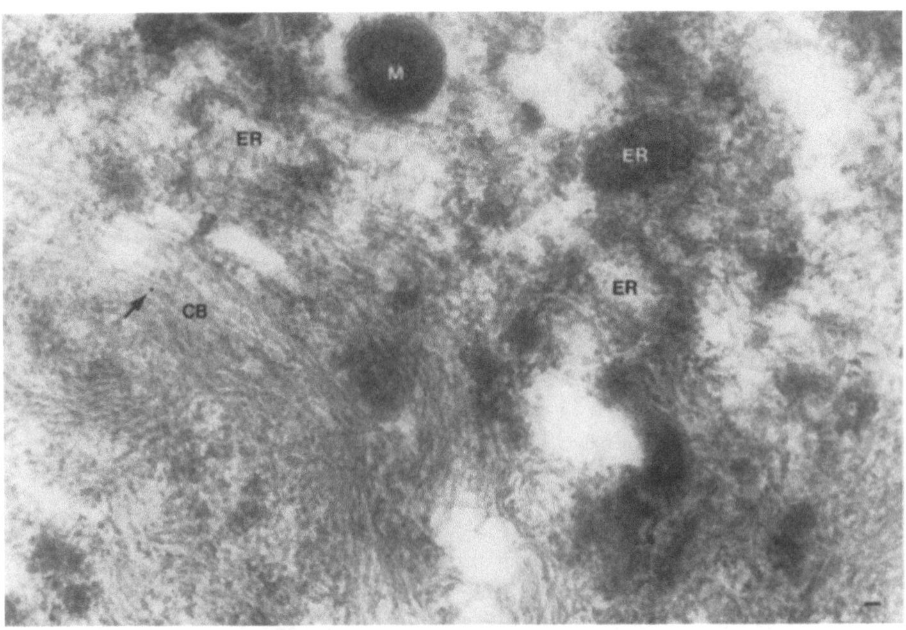

Fig. 4. Frozen sections of human fibroblasts in culture show only negligible gold particles (*arrow*) after performing the same labelling procedure as used in Figs. 1–3. *CB*, Collagen bundle; *ER*, endoplasmic reticulum; *M*, mitochondrium. *Bar*, 0.5 μm

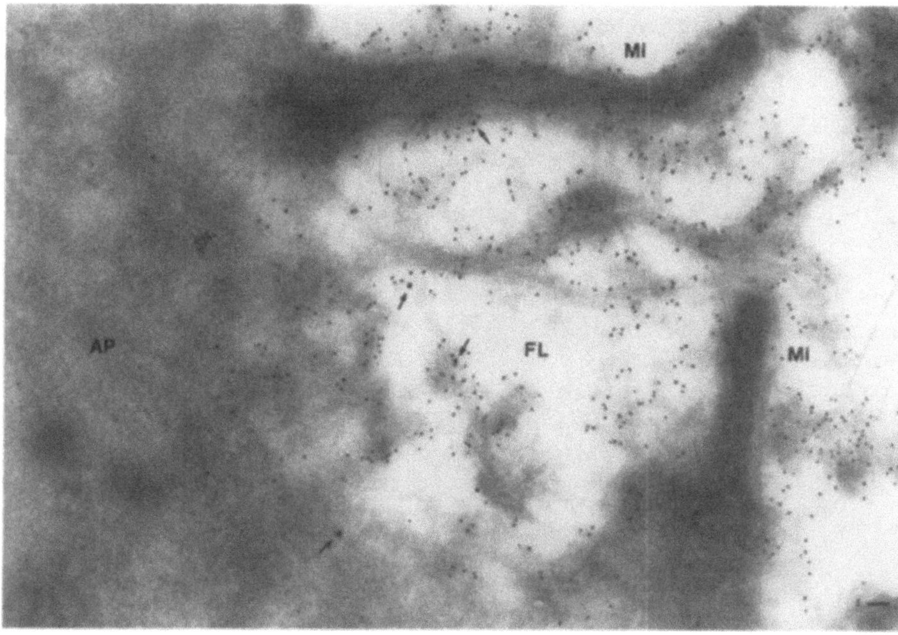

Fig. 5. Frozen sections of a follicle obtained from patient 3 is labelled with biotinylated rabbit $F(ab')_2$ fragments against the Fc_γ fragment of human IgG (gold particles with a diameter of 10 nm) and an antibody against thyroglobulin (gold particles with a diameter of 6 nm). There are only a few IgG (arrows) located in the follicular lumen (*FL*), in contrast to the high amount of thyroglobulin. *AP*, Apical pole; *Mi*, microvilli. *Bar*, 0.5 μm

In order to estimate the concentration of IgG at the luminal site of follicular cells, we assessed the number of gold particles labelling biotinylated $F(ab')_2$ fragments against the human γ chain/μm^2 section of 10 mg IgG per millilitre of gelatine. This dilution corresponded to the concentration of IgG in normal human serum. Comparing the labelling densities of different sizes of gold particles (sections of 10 mg IgA/ml gelatine as control), our results showed labelling of 10 mg IgG/ml gelatine by streptavidin gold of 5 nm diameter at a density of approximately 10 gold particles/μm^2 and by streptavidin gold of 10 nm diameter at a density of approximately 2 gold particles/μm^2 (Fig. 7). The labelling density was about 20 times lower when the antibody against IgG and streptavidin gold 10 nm was applied on sections of 10 mg IgA/ml gelatine.

4 Discussion

Due to the fact that surface expression of TPO is restricted to the apical membrane of follicular cells in the normal thyroid gland and that autoantibodies against TPO play a major role in thyroid autoimmunity, it is an important question whether IgG

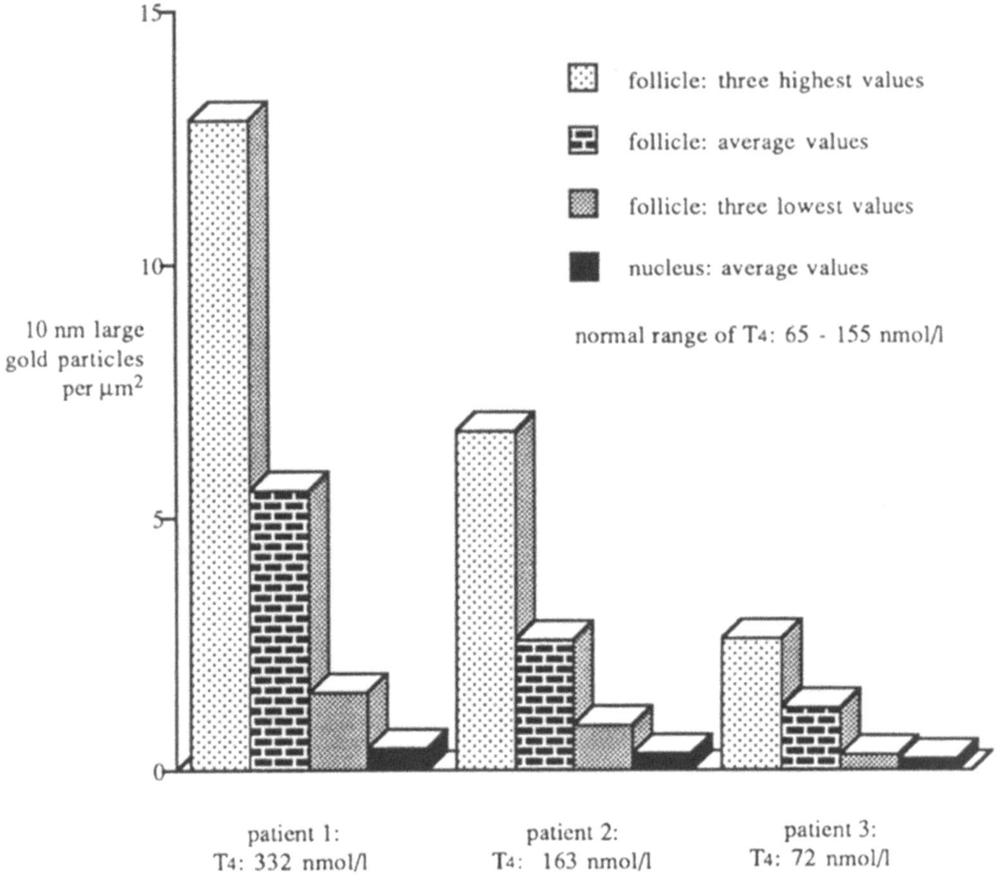

Fig. 6. The labelling density of IgG over the follicular lumina of three patients is indicated by the number of 10 nm large gold particles per square micrometre (maximum, average and minimum values for each patient). The low amount of labelling over the nucleus reveals the specificity of the labelling procedure. The amount of IgG measured in the follicular lumina is higher in the hyperthyroid patients in comparison to the euthyroid patient

can be located in vivo on the apical surface of follicular cells in patients with autoimmune thyroiditis. The detection by direct immunofluorescence of IgG in thyroid gland of patients suffering from autoimmune thyroiditis has produced nonconclusive results. While most studies were unable to demonstrate the presence of IgG on the apical membrane (Werner et al. 1972; Kalderon and Bogaars 1977; Fujiwara et al. 1981; Okamoto et al. 1991), others have described deposits of IgG delineating the apical border of the follicular epithelium (Koffler and Friedman 1963; Khoury et al. 1984). Our results confirm that in follicular cells in autoimmune thyroiditis, IgG is specifically located close to the luminal face of the apical membrane. Several control experiments have proved the specificity of this labelling. In our studies the labelling density of IgG in the follicular lumina

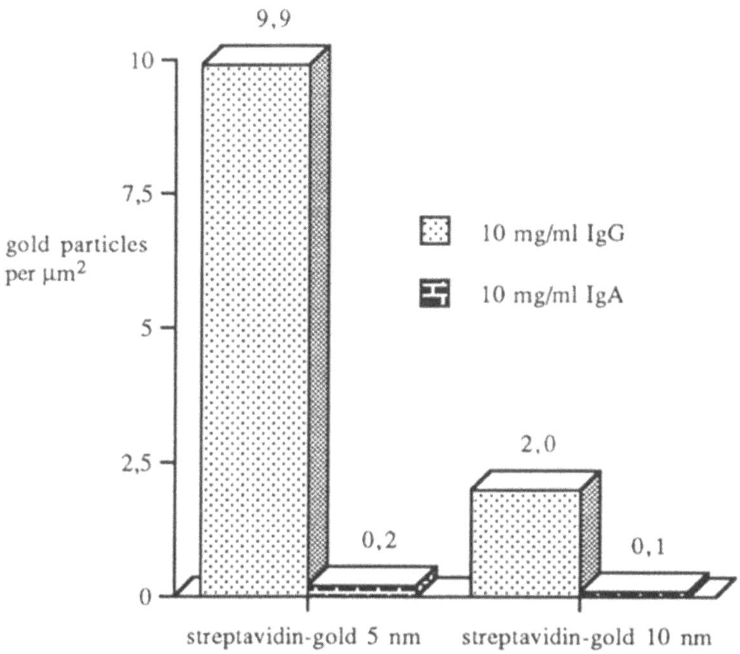

Fig. 7. The number of gold particles per square micrometre of area were determined on thin frozen sections of IgG embedded in gelatine at a concentration of 64 mg/ml using biotinylated rabbit $F(ab')_2$ fragments against the Fc_γ fragment of human IgG. Streptavidin gold with a diameter of 5 nm indicates about five times as many IgG molecules as streptavidin gold with a diameter of 10 nm. This antibody labels IgA to a much lesser extent, at least 20 times lower than IgG

varied considerably. Quantitative evaluation of the IgG labelling revealed a maximum concentration of IgG inside the follicular lumina of 64 mg/ml. Most of the IgG molecules were located close to the apical membrane and, to a much lesser degree, in the centre of the follicular lumina. This labelling pattern suggests that the labelled IgG is directed against TPO. This is supported by co-localising IgG and TG, which showed only a few IgG molecules in areas with TG accumulation.

Studying the pathogenetic role of IgG in vivo, it was intriguing to see that IgG located in the extracellular space is only in contact to the basolateral surface of thyrocytes. By what pathway(s) is IgG transported from the basolateral to the apical membrane? First, it is unlikely that IgG approaches the apical membrane of thyrocytes directly from the extracellular space through tight junctions of the polarized cells, because macromolecules such as IgG (200 Å) have not been reported to pass tight junctions. At present, tight junctions are considered to be an effective seal for molecules measuring 11.5 Å or greater in Stokes radius. Fragmentation of tight junctions, as described in certain disease states and experimental intestinal cell systems (MADARA 1989), has been observed only exceptionally in diseased thyroid gland, and has not been noticed in normal thyroid gland (HEIMANN 1966). Additionally, destruction or breakdown of thyroid follicles is more probably the consequence than the initiation of the thyroid autoimmune process. Secondly, molecules from the extracellular space can be imported into the cell's interior by receptor-mediated endocytosis (ligands), pinocytosis (fluid), phagocytosis (particles such as viruses and bacteria) and membrane channels (e.g., glucose). IgG as a macromolecule is known to be endocytosed by cells bearing the Fc receptor, such as macrophages (RAVETCH and KINET 1991). This receptor has not been detected on thyrocytes. Thirdly, transcytosis of immunoglobulins across polarised cells, which has been described in enterocytes (IgA and IgM), intestinal epithelium in newborn rats (IgG) and human placenta (IgG) (MOSTOV 1991), has not been observed in the thyroid gland. The only transcytosis established in thyrocytes is the biosynthetic pathway of thyroglobulin (ROMAGNOLI and HERZOG 1991). The mechanism of receptor-mediated transcytosis is well characterised in Madin-Darby canine kidney (MDCK) cells transfected with the polymeric IgA receptor. This receptor transfers IgA by a multi-step vesicular transport from the basolateral to the apical plasma membrane. Early endosomes originating from the basolateral membrane deliver IgA by means of transcytotic vesicles to an apically located endosomal compartment, where IgA is translocated to the apical lumen by a brefeldin- and G-protein-sensitive mechanism (BARROSO and SZTUL 1994). Since we observed IgG in intracellular vesicles of thyrocytes (Fig. 2), it may be suggested that transcytosis is responsible for the transport of IgG from the basolateral to the apical membrane in thyrocytes of patients with autoimmune thyroiditis.

Although we have evidence that IgG reaches the follicular lumen by transcytotic transport vesicles, it is unclear by which receptor IgG is bound on the basolateral membrane and how its translocation to the apical membrane is mediated. We suppose that this receptor is related to the protein which initiates the antigen presentation in thyroid autoimmunity. Therefore the question arises how a membrane protein like TPO, which is restricted to the apical membrane, is presented to T lymphocytes in order to produce antibodies against it. Two mechanisms may be involved in these processes: (a) antibodies with dual specificity against TG and TPO and (b) mis-sorting of TPO to the basolateral membrane. There is evidence that autoantibodies from patients with autoimmune thyroiditis cross-react with TG and TPO (KOHNO et al. 1988; RUF et al. 1992). Since TG as a secretory protein has no receptor function, the existence of antibodies with dual specificity against TG and TPO does not explain how autoantibodies can be transcytosed from the basolateral to the apical membrane of thyrocytes. On the other hand, mis-sorted TPO molecules or reversal of thyrocyte polarity could be responsible for the initiation of antigen presentation as well as the uptake of autoantibodies from the basolateral membrane. While reversal of thyroid epithelial polarity has already been reported (HANAFUSA et al. 1984), there are no data supporting mis-sorting of TPO. In the light of our qualitative examinations, the amount of TPO on the basolateral membrane of thyrocytes seems to be negligible (ZIMMER et al. 1992). It is necessary to quantify the amount of TPO on the apical membrane in comparison to the basolateral membrane of patients with autoimmune thyroid disease and control thyroid tissue. Because mutations in the signal sequence of TPO may cause mis-sorting, it seems worthwhile to search for somatic point mutations in the TPO gene of patients with autoimmune disease. Recently, a mutation in a putative ligand-binding domain of the TSH receptor has been described in a patient with Graves' disease (HELDIN et al. 1991).

References

Banga JP, Barnett PS, McGregor AM (1991) Immunological and molecular characteristics of the thyroid peroxidase autoantigen. Autoimmunity 8: 335–343

Barroso M, Sztul E (1994) Basolateral to apical transcytosis in polarized cells is indirect and involves BFA and trimeric G protein sensitive passage through the apical endosome. J Cell Biol 124: 83–100

Bogner U, Schleusener H, Wall JR (1984) Antibody-dependent cell mediated cytotoxicity against human thyroid cells in Hashimoto's thyroiditis but not Graves' disease. J Clin Endocrinol Metab 59: 734–738

Braciale TJ, Braciale VL (1991) Antigen presentation: structural themes and functional variations. Immunol Today 12: 124–129

Chazenbalk GD, Portolano S, Russo D, Hutchison JS, Rapoport B, McLachlan S (1993) Human organ-specific autoimmune disease. Molecular cloning and expression of an autoantibody gene repertoire for a major autoantigen reveals an antigenic immunodominant region and restricted immunoglobulin gene usage in the target organ. J Clin Invest 92: 62–74

Copeland C, Zimmer KP, Wagner KR, Healey GA, Mellman I, Helenius A (1988) Folding, trimerization, and transport are sequential events in the biogenesis of influenza virus hemagglutinin. Cell 53: 197–209

Davies TF, Martin A, Concepcion ES, Graves P, Cohen L, Ben-Nun A (1991) Evidence of limited variability of antigen receptors on intrathyroidal T cells in autoimmune thyroid disease. N Engl J Med 325: 238–244

Fujiwara H, Forisu M, Sugisaki T, Okano H (1981) Immune complex deposits in thyroid glands of patients with Graves' disease. II. Anti-thyroglobulin and anti-microsomal activities of γ-globulin eluted from thyroid homogenates. Clin Immunol Immunopathol 19: 109–117

Griffiths G (1993) Fine structure immunocytochemistry. Springer, Berlin Heidelberg New York

Hanafusa T, Pujol-Borrell R, Chiovato L, Doniach D, Bottazzo GF (1984) In vitro and in vivo reversal of thyroid epithelial polarity: its relevance for autoimmune thyroid disease. Clin Exp Immunol 58: 639–646

Heimann P (1966) Ultrastructure of human thyroid. Acta Endocrinol (Copenh) 53 Suppl 110: 3–102

Heldin NE, Gustavsson B, Westermark K, Westermark B (1991) A somatic point mutation in a putative ligand binding domain of the TSH receptor in a patient with autoimmune hyperthyroidism. J Clin Endocrinol Metab 73: 1374–1376

Henry M, Zanelli E, Piechaczyk M, Pau B, Malthièry Y (1992) A major human thyroglobulin epitope defined with monoclonal antibodies is mainly recognized by human autoantibodies. Eur J Immunol 22: 315–319

Kalderon AE, Bogaars HA (1977) Immune complex deposits in Graves' disease and Hashimoto's thyroiditis. Am J Med 63: 729–734

Khoury EL, Hammond L, Bottazzo GF, Doniach D (1981) Presence of the organ-specific "microsomal" autoantigen on the surface of human thyroid cells in culture: its involvement in complement-mediated cytotoxicity. Clin Exp Immunol 45: 316–328

Khoury EL, Bottazzo GF, Roitt IM (1984) The thyroid "microsomal" antibody revisited. Its paradoxical binding in vivo to the apical surface of the follicular epithelium. J Exp Med 159: 577–591

Kimura S, Kotani T, McBride OW, Umeki K, Hirai K, Nakayama T, Ohtaki S (1987) Human thyroid peroxidase: complete cDNA and protein sequence, chromosome mapping, and identification of two alternately spliced mRNAs. Proc Natl Acad Sci USA 84: 5555–5559

Koffler D, Friedman AH (1964) Localization of immunoglobulins in chronic thyroiditis. Lab Invest 13: 239–245

Kohno Y, Naito N, Hiyama Y, Shimojo N, Suzuki N, Tarutani O, Niimi H, Nakajima H, Hosoya T (1988) Thyroglobulin and thyroid peroxidase share common epitopes recognized by autoantibodies in patients with chronic autoimmune thyroiditis. J Clin Endocrinol Metab 67: 899–907

Kohno Y, Yamaguchi F, Saito K, Niimi H, Nishikawa T, Hosoya T (1991) Anti-thyroid peroxidase antibodies in sera from healthy subjects and from patients with chronic thyroiditis: differences in the ability to inhibit thyroid peroxidase activities. Clin Exp Immunol 85: 459–463

Libert F, Ruel J, Lugdate M, Swillens S, Alexander N, Vassart G, Dinsart C (1987) Thyroperoxidase, an auto-antigen with a mosaic structure made of nuclear and mitochondrial gene modules. EMBO J 6: 4193–4196

Libert F, Lefort A, Gerard C, Parmentier M, Perret J, Ludgate M, Dumont JE, Vassart G (1989) Cloning, sequencing and expression of the human thyrotropin (TSH) receptor: evidence for binding of autoantibodies. Biochem Biophys Res Commun 165: 1250–1255

Madara JL (1989) Loosening tight junctions. J Clin Invest 83: 1089–1094

Malthièry Y, Lissitzky S (1987) Primary structure of human thyroglobulin deduced from the sequence of its 8448-base complementary DNA. Eur J Biochem 165: 491–498

Mostov K (1991) The polymeric immunoglobulin receptor. Sem in Cell Biol 2: 411–418

Nagayama Y, Rapoport B (1992) The thyrotropin receptor 25 years after its discovery: new insight after its molecular cloning. Mol Endocrinol 6: 145–156

Nagayama Y, Kaufman KD, Seto P, Rapoport B (1989) Molecular cloning, sequence and functional expression of the cDNA for the human thyrotropin receptor. Biochem Biophys Res Commun 165: 1184–1190

Nunez J, Pommier J (1982) Formation of thyroid hormones. Vitam Horm 39: 175–229

Okamoto Y, Hamada N, Saito H, Ohno M, Noh J, Ito K, Morii H (1989) Thyroid peroxidase activity-inhibiting immunoglobulins in patients with autoimmune thyroid disease. J Clin Endocrinol Metabol 68: 730–734

Okamoto Y, Hamada N, Fujisawa T, Noh J, Yamakawa J, Ohno M, Ito K, Morii H (1991) Why no simple relationship between thyroid peroxidase activity-inhibiting immunoglobulins and thyroid function in autoimmune thyroid disease? Acta Endocrinol (copenh) 124: 442–448

Pinchera A, Mariotti S, Vitti P, Marcocci C, Chivatto L, Fenzi G, Santini F (1989) Thyroid autoantigens and their relevance in the pathogenesis of thyroid autoimmunity. Biochimie 71: 237–245

Ravetch JV, Kinet JP (1991) Fc receptors. Annu Rev Immunol 9: 457–492

Romagnoli P, Herzog V (1991) Transcytosis in thyroid follicle cells: regulation and implications for thyroglobulin transport. Exp Cell Res 194: 202–209

Ruf J, Ferrand M, Durand-Gorde JM, Carayon P (1992) Immunopurification and characterization of thyroid autoantibodies with dual specificity for thyroglobulin and thyroperoxidase. Autoimmunity 11: 179–188

Saller B, Hörmann R, Mann K (1991) Heterogeneity of autoantibodies against thyroid peroxidase in autoimmune thyroid disease: evidence against antibodies directly inhibiting peroxidase activity as regulatory factors in thyroid hormone metabolism. J Clin Endocrinol Metab 72: 188–195

Schulz E, Benker G, Bethäuser H, Stempka L, Hüfer M (1992) An autoimmuno-dominant thyroglobulin epitope characterized by a monoclonal antibody. J Endocrinol Invest 15: 25–30

Slot JW, Geuze HJ (1985) A new method of preparing gold probes for multiple-labeling cytochemistry. Eur J Cell Biol 38: 87–93

Strakvosch CR, Wenzel BE, Row VV, Volpe R (1982) Immunology of autoimmune thyroid diseases. N Engl J Med 307: 1499–1507

Taurog A (1986) Hormone synthesis: thyroid iodine metabolism. In: Ingbar SH, Braverman LE (eds) Werner's the thyroid, 5th edn. Lippincott, Philadelphia, pp 53–97

Utiger (1991) The pathogenesis of autoimmune thyroid disease. N Engl J Med: 325: 278–279

Werner SC, Wegelius O, Fierer JA, Hsu KC (1972) Immunoglobulins (E, M, G) and complement in the connective tissues of the thyroid in Graves' disease. N Engl J Med 287: 421–425

Zakarija M, McKenzie JM (1987) The spectrum and significance of autoantibodies reacting with the thyrotropin receptor. Endocrinol Metab Clin North Am 16: 343–363

Zimmer KP, Hengst K, Carayon P, Brämswig J, Harms E (1992) Different concentrations of thyroid peroxidase and thyroglobulin in the nuclear envelope and the endoplasmic reticulum throughout the cytoplasm. Eur J Cell Biol 57: 12–20

Clinical Aspects and Diagnosis of Thyroid Hormone Transport Protein Anomalies

W. Langsteger

Current Topics in Pathology
Volume 91, K.W. Schmid/W. Böcker (Eds.)

1 Introduction

The thyroid hormones T_4 (thyroxine) and T_3 (3,5,3′-triiodothyronine) circulate in the blood reversibly bound to proteins. The principal transport proteins are: T_4-binding globulin (TBG), transthyretin (TTR), formerly called T_4-binding prealbumin or TBPA, and albumin. These proteins differ widely in concentration and their affinity for the iodothyronines (OPPENHEIMER 1968; ROBBINS and RALL 1960; ROBBINS et al. 1986); collectively, they carry more than 99% of T_3 and T_4 in serum. Other thyroid hormone-binding proteins in serum are lipoproteins (BENVENGA 1989; BENVENGA et al. 1988, 1989, 1990), for example the 27 K protein, an apolipoprotein A–I, and the apolipoprotein B-100, which are both synthesized in the liver (GRIMALDI et al. 1986; BARTALENA et al. 1986a,b). Less important binding proteins are immunoglobulin M (SVIRIDOV et al. 1991) and, in thyroid autoimmune disorders, thyroid hormone autoantibodies of the IgG class (BENVENGA et al. 1987).

The main function of thyroid hormone transport serum proteins is the extrathyroidal storage of T_4 and T_3, buffering acute changes in thyroid hormone secretion and thus providing a more constant delivery of the hormones to target tissues (DOCTER et al. 1984; ROBBINS 1991). Thyroid hormone transport proteins, following interactions with specific receptors on the cell surface, also play a role in hormone entry: TBG in peripheral mononuclear cells (HASHIZUME et al. 1986), TTR in astrocytoma and liver cells (DIVINO and SCHUSSLER 1989, 1990) and lipoproteins in human fibroblasts (BENVENGA and ROBBINS 1990; BARTALENA and ROBBINS 1992). Furthermore, a role of TBG in the uniform cellular distribution of thyroid hormones has also been suggested (MENDEL et al. 1987).

Variations of thyroid hormone-binding protein may be acquired or genetically determined and may involve changes in their quantity or their affinity for thyroid hormones. Such alterations can be associated with substantial changes in the thyroid hormone-binding capacity of serum. While abnormalities most frequently involve TBG, changes in albumin and TTR are being recognized with increased frequency.

2 T_4-Binding Globulin

Native or common-type TBG (TBG-C), a 54-kDa glycoprotein of hepatic origin (GORDON et al. 1952; GERSHENGORN et al. 1977; HOCHMAN 1981; BARTALENA and ROBBINS 1984; MURATA et al. 1985), is the major thyroid hormone carrier protein in human serum (REFETOFF 1979a). Cloning and sequencing of human TBG has shown that TBG is synthesized as a 415-amino-acid protein with a high degree of homology; surprisingly, it shows also great homology (55%) with corticosteroid-binding-globulin (CBG) (FLINK et al. 1986; HAMMOND et al. 1987; JANSSEN et al. 1992). TBG has only one binding site for T_4 and T_3, and binds T_4 with higher affinity than T_3; furthermore, the noncovalent T_4 binding to TBG stabilizes the molecule (GRIMALDI and ROBBINS 1982). Details of physicochemical properties and binding characteristics (CAVALIERI et al. 1975; REFETOFF et al. 1975) are shown in Tables 1–4.

Table 1. Physico-chemical properties of thyroid hormones

	Bound (%)	Free (%)	$t_{1/2}$	Production rate (μg/day)	Biological activity
Thyroxine (T_4)	99.97	0.03	7 days	100	100
Tri-iodo-thyronine (T_3)	99.7	0.3	20 h	10	300–800
Reverse T_3 (rT_3)			4–5 h	1	<1

Table 2. Binding characteristics and physico-chemical properties of thyroid hormone transport proteins

	mw	T_4 binding (%)	T_3 binding (%)	Synthesis	$t_{1/2}$
TBG-C (single-chain glycoprotein)	54 kDa	70–75	65–70	Liver	5 days
Albumin (single chain)	66 kDa	20	10–35	Liver	
TTR (tetramer; four subunits)	55 kDa	10–15	<1	Liver, CNS, pancreas	2.5 days

TBG, T_4-binding globulin; TTR, transthyretin.

Table 3. Binding characteristics of thyroid hormone transport proteins (normal serum, 37°C, physiological pH)

	Affinity K_a (M^{-1})	Capacity (mg T_4/100 ml serum)	Concentration (mg/dl)	Production rate (mg/day per 70 kg)
TBG	1.0×10^{10}	20	1.5–3.0	13–18
Albumin	7.0×10^{5}	>800	4200	14000
TTR	7.0×10^{7}	300	12–25	510–680

The basic question of the role played by the TBG has to be discussed (Ingbar 1961; Refetoff et al. 1976; Robbins et al. 1978; Gärtner et al. 1981), since TBG deficiency is not accompanied by any alteration of the production of thyroid hormones or by an altered metabolic status of the organism (Robbins 1973; Refetoff and Larsen 1989). There is reason to believe that TBG has multiple functions, namely:

- Avoidance of iodine loss through urine excretion (Chan et al. 1972)
- Improvement of cellular T_4 distribution to achieve faster cellular response (Mendel et al. 1987)
- Termination of the delivery of thyroid hormones after reaching of the desired levels – at present a rather hypothetical function (Pemberton et al. 1988)

Table 4. Detailed binding characteristics of T_4 and T_3 (normal serum, 37°C, physiological pH)

		T_4		T_3	
		Affinity constant (M^{-1})	Dissociation rate $t_{1/2}$ (s)	Affinity constant (M^{-1})	Dissociation rate $t_{1/2}$ (s)
TBG		1.0×10^{10}	39	5.0×10^{8}	4
Albumin:	site 1	7.0×10^{5}	<1	1.0×10^{5}	<1
	site 2–6	5.0×10^{4}		5.0×10^{3}	
TTR:	site 1	7.0×10^{7}	7.4	1.0×10^{7}	1
	site 2	7.0×10^{5}		6.0×10^{5}	

- Above all, protection of the organism when sudden changes occur in the hormonal and metabolic situation (e.g. during pregnancy an increase in TBG to provide a "buffer" store is observed) (REFETOFF 1989).

Although TBG is not essential for thyroid hormone action, alterations in its concentration produce proportional changes in the levels of circulation T_4 and T_3 (REFETOFF 1979a; ROBBINS and BARTALENA 1986). Familial X-linked total and partial TBG deficiency and TBG variants with decreased affinity for T_4 have been described (ROBBINS and BARTALENA 1986; REFETOFF 1989; MORI et al. 1988); all the subjects are euthyroid, have normal survival rates and have no detectable difficulties or handicaps (ROBBINS and RALL 1960; OPPENHEIMER 1968; REFETOFF et al. 1972; REFETOFF 1979a; BURR et al. 1980; BARTALENA and ROBBINS 1984; MURATA et al. 1985; REFETOFF and MURATA 1985).

2.1 Inherited Variants of TBG

Inherited abnormalities of the TBG concentration (Tables 5, 6) include complete deficiency (TBG-CD), partial deficiency (TBG-PD) and TBG excess (TBG-X). They are encountered amongst all ethnic groups and races investigated (REFETOFF 1979a; REFETOFF et al. 1972; BURR et al. 1980). These defects have an X-chromosome-linked mode of inheritance (REFETOFF and LARSEN 1989; REFETOFF et al. 1972; BURR et al. 1980), in agreement with the localization of the single TBG gene copy to the long arm of the X chromosome (TRENT et al. 1987). The mechanisms responsible for these defects include nucleotide deletions (YAMAMORI et al. 1991; LI et al. 1991) and amino acid substitutions (MORI et al. 1990; JANSSEN et al. 1991; TAKEDA et al. 1989; WALTZ et al. 1990; BERTENSHAW 1991).

TBG deficiency is rarely associated with a functional thyroid disorder (Table 7), and consequently studying the secretion and metabolism of thyroid hormones is of little value in such cases. TBG deficiency has been found in association with both hyperthyroidism (BURR et al. 1980; KAMIKUBO et al. 1985; ISHIZUKI et al. 1981; NAKAGAWA et al. 1967; STRUNGE 1974; GERSTNER and KAPLAN 1976; HORWITZ and REFETOFF 1977; YABU et al. 1980) and hypothyroidism (HANSTED and MOLLER 1984; NIKOLAI and SEAL 1966; MOLOSHOK et al. 1969). Albumin and

Table 5. Inherited variants of thyroid hormone transport proteins

	Concentration			Affinity		Poly-morphism
	Excess	Deficiency	Absence	Increased	Decreased	
TBG (X-linked)	X	X	X	–	X	X
Albumin (autosomal dominant)	–	–	X	X	–	X
TTR (autosomal dominant)	–	?	–	X	X	X

Table 6. Inherited variants of thyroid hormone transport proteins

	Concentration		Affinity		
	Excess	Deficiency	Absence	Increased	Decreased
TBG (X-linked)	TBG-X (1:40000)	TBG-PD (1:4000)	TBG-CD (1:15000)	–	X
Albumin (autosomal dominant)	–	–	An-albuminaemia	FDH 1:10000 type I–IV	–
TTR (autosomal dominant)	–	?	–	TTR-AH (PAAH) type I–II	FAP

X, Excess; PD, partial deficiency; CD, complete deficiency; FDH, familial dysalbuminaemic hyperthyroxinaemia; TTR-AH, transthyretin-associated hyperthyroxinaemia; PAAH, prealbumin-associated hyperthyroxinaemia.

Table 7. Thyroid disorders (11) in individuals with variant transport proteins

TBG-PD:	Hyperthyroidism (4) NAKAGAWA et al. (1967) Hypothyroidism (1) HANSTED et al. (1984)
FDH:	Hyperthyroidism (3) CROXSON et al. (1985) Hypothyroidism (1) YOUNG et al. (1987) Post-partum thyroiditis (1) LANGSTEGER et al. (1994)

PA were normal in all of these cases, and the TBG deficiency was not detectable by radioimmunoassay methods. Nevertheless, because of inappropriate testing and erroneous diagnosis, subjects with TBG-X have been treated for thyrotoxicosis (MOLOSHOK et al. 1969; LEAHY et al. 1984), and subjects with TBG deficiency have received T_4 medication for hypothyroidism (REFETOFF and SELENKOW 1968; SARNE et al. 1989).

Finally, the possibility that TBG deficiency prevents the transmission of familial dysalbuminemic hyperthyroxinemia (FDH) remains a matter of speculation (LANGSTEGER et al. 1994).

Complete TBG deficiency is defined by a TBG serum concentration limit of 0.005 mg/l, corresponding to about 0.03% of the average TBG concentration in the serum of adults. TBG-CD occurs in 1 in 15000 newborn males (COPPING and BYFIELD 1988) and has no racial or ethnic preponderances (JENKINS and STEFFES 1987).

Partial TBG deficiency occurs in approximately 1 in 4000 (REFETOFF 1989). Two of the first TBG variants discovered, characterized by reduced serum TBG concentrations (DAIGER et al. 1981; REFETOFF and MURATA 1985) *and* reduced affinity for T_4 or T_3, should be mentioned:

(i) TBG-A (aborigines), only found among the Australian aborigines with a prevalence of about 40% (MURATA et al. 1985; DICK and WATSON 1981), is characterized by a normal isoelectric focusing (IEF) pattern, a reduced affinity for T_4 and T_3, and an increased susceptibility to inactivation by heat or acid. The cause is a structural defect of the TBG polypeptide chain: double amino acid substitution in position 191 (Ala – Thr) and in position 283 (Leu – Phe), a finding confirmed by TAKAMATSU et al. in 1987. The case published by MURATA et al. in 1986 is also to be regarded primarily as a TBG-A variant.

(ii) TBG-S (slow), confined to blacks, Eskimos, Melanesians, Polynesians and Indonesians (DAIGER et al. 1981; KAMBOH and KIRWOOD 1984), among whom it has a prevalence of about 5%–10%, was first described by DAIGER et al. in 1981: single amino acid substitution in position 171 (Asp – Asn). It exhibits a cathodal shift in isoelectric focusing (TAKAMATSU et al. 1986; DAIGER et al. 1981); occupation of the thyroxine-binding site stabilizes the molecule and protects it against denaturation by heat (REFETOFF et al. 1984; GRIMALDI et al. 1982). The spontaneous disappearance rate of this native TBG variant in serum at 37°C, with an initial half-life of 3h, is at least 40 times as fast as the turnover rate of normal native TBG (GRIMALDI et al. 1983).

TBG excess, probably related to changes in the regulatory sequences of the TBG gene promoter (BARTALENA and ROBBINS 1992), occurs at a prevalence of 1 in 6000 to 1 in 40000 (BROWN and BELLISARIO 1986; LYON 1983; GRIFFITHS et al. 1985).

2.2 Acquired Variants of TGB

Acquired abnormalities of TGB, caused by stimulation or inhibition of TBG synthesis (Table 8), are associated with a variety of drugs and pathophysiologic con-

Table 8. Causes of acquired variants of TBG

Serum concentration of TBG	
Increased	Decreased
Pregnancy	Malnutrition
Liver disorders	Nephrotic syndrome
AIDS	Acromegaly
Drugs: Heroin	Drugs: Androgens
Methadone	Glucocorticoids
5-Fluorouracil	Anabolic steroids
Clofibrate	
Oestrogens	

ditions (Robbins and Bartalena 1986; Bartalena 1990). They may be caused extrathyroidally by pregnancy, liver disorders (Robbins and Bartalena 1986; Ain and Refetoff 1988), AIDS (LoPresti et al. 1989; Lambert et al. 1990), malnutrition and nephrotic syndromes. Drugs affecting serum TBG concentrations include IL-6, heroin, methadone, clofibrate, 5-FU and L-asparaginase, as well as oestrogens (Bartalena 1990; Glinoer et al. 1977), androgens and glucocorticoid excess (Kamikubo et al. 1985; Whitecar et al. 1970; Bartalena et al. 1986). The most important acquired variations of TGB will be discussed now in more detail.

2.2.1 Acquired Immune Deficiency Syndrome (AIDS)

Syndromes of acquired immundeficiency show variations in thyroid function tests: serum total T_4 (TT4) values are normal or elevated, serum total T_3 (TT3) concentrations are normal and serum rT_3 levels are normal or low (LoPresti et al. 1989). Increased serum TBG levels – possible due to increased liver synthesis of the protein – are found especially in patients with advanced disease (Refetoff and Larsen 1989), but changes in sialylation of TBG are a possibility. The lack of concomitant changes in serum SHBG is important in the differential diagnosis of the classic low-T_3 syndrome associated with nonthyroidal illness.

2.2.2 Liver Disorders

In patients with acute and chronic hepatitis, and also in many patients with hepatocellular carcinoma (HCC), increased serum TBG levels were estimated (Robbins and Bartalena 1986). The increase in serum TBG concentration seems to be a result of increased synthesis after hepatocellular damage (Huang and Liaw 1990), but the mechanisms leading to these changes are unclear. This thesis would be supported by the fact that serum TBG concentrations are moderately increased in patients with liver cirrhosis who do not develop HCC, but increase progressively in HCC patients (Alexopoulos et al. 1988).

2.2.3 Pregnancy

The increase of TBG in pregnancy seems to be related to a physiological role of TBG in the delivery of thyroid hormones to the fetoplacental unit, which is essential for normal fetal development (EKINS et al. 1989). This seems to be supported by the observation that lower serum TBG concentrations than normal are associated with an increased risk of abortion or lower birth weight, or even increased occurrence of fetal malformation (ROSS et al. 1989; LAO et al. 1989; SPARRE 1989). The increase in TBG synthesis is caused by an oestrogen-induced synthesis increase in the liver (ROBBINS and BARTALENA 1986); however, it was shown by AIN et al. (1987) that TBG in the serum of pregnant women is more heavily sialylated and also has a longer half-life than normal TBG.

2.3 Thyroid Function Parameters

Because of an increase in both peripheral conversion of TT_4 to TT_3 (ABUID and LARSEN 1974; AMINO et al. 1981; INADA et al. 1975) and thyroid excretion of TT_3 (LARSEN 1972), TT_4 or FT_4 values are far lower than T_3 values in individuals with TBG deficiency (KAMIKUBO et al. 1985). Peculiarly enough, the high affinity of T_4 to TBG and the high specifity of the binding does not seem to have any significant physiological function (REFETOFF et al. 1984), as demonstrated by the fact that, for example, TBG-CD does not lead to hypothyroidism (REFETOFF 1989; TANAKA and STARR 1959). Only the oestrogen-induced increase in TBG seems to serve a physiological purpose, namely, improved transfer of T_4 between mother and fetus (SCHUSSLER 1990).

3 Albumin

Albumin is a 66-kDa protein, has one major binding site for T_4, consists of one polypeptide chain and is synthesized in the liver (HENNEMANN and DOCTER 1990; PETERS 1975). For details of its physico-chemical properties and binding characteristics see Tables 2–4.

The most common cause of variants of albumin (Tables 5, 6) in euthyroid hyperthyroxinaemia is the familial dysalbuminaemic hyperthyroxinaemia (FDH) syndrome (STOCKIGT et al. 1981; LALLOZ et al. 1983, 1986; YABU et al. 1985; DIVINO and SCHUSSLER 1990). Findings of albumin being the abnormal T_4-binding protein in FDH are based on different detection methods, such as electrophoresis, sepharose chromatography (WEISS et al. 1995; DOCTER et al. 1981; BARLOW et al. 1986), T_4 precipitation with albumin antisera (STOCKIGT et al. 1981, 1983; WEISS et al. 1995; TAKAMATSU and OHSAWA 1990) and, finally, by modified gel electrophoretic methods (WAKONIG et al. 1987; LANGSTEGER et al. 1994a), which are described in more detail in Sect. 5.

Sera of FDH subjects contain normal and FDH albumin (Schussler 1990). Isoelectric focusing (IEF) has shown that in normal albumin, radioiodinated T_4 mostly binds to ph 5.44 and 5.31 and, to a lower extent, to ph 5.22 and 4.79 (Yabu et al. 1985). The FDH albumin may be a protein that has properties in common with albumin and cross-reacts with albumin antisera (Weiss et al. 1995), because most T_4 is bound to bands ph 5.22 and 4.79 (Yabu et al. 1985; Docter et al. 1981). The high T_4 binding to serum protein could come about by abnormal processing of mRNA of albumin (Weiss et al. 1995). Nevertheless, FDH patients have also been seen without any differences in albumin (Yabu et al. 1985). These facts should be kept in mind when interpreting IEF of T_4-binding in the presence of low pH (Divino and Schussler 1990).

It has also been suggested that the increased affinity and specificity of the variant albumin for thyroid hormone may be due to an electrostatic interaction between the ionized phenolic hydroxyl of the iodothyronine and a cationic group on the protein (Divino and Schussler 1989), affecting electrophoretic mobility (Rushebrook et al. 1995); in FDH, studies of T_4 kinetics have shown both normal and increased T_4 disposal rates (Mendel and Cavalieri 1984; Bianchi et al. 1987).

3.1 Inherited Albumin Variants

FDH, also called albumin-associated hyperthyroxinaemia (AAH), familial euthyroid thyroxine excess, congenital thyroxine-binding albumin elevation, or euthyroid isolated hyperthyroxinaemia, was first described by Hennemann et al. (1979) and by Lee et al. in 1979. It is characterized by the presence of a variant albumin-like protein with an increased affinity for iodothyronines (Bartalena 1990), and has an autosomal dominant inheritance pattern. The prevalence (Table 6) ranges from 1 in 50 (DeCosimo et al. 1987) to approximately 1 in 10000 subjects (Jensen et al. 1990; Jensen and Faber 1988), and depends also on the ethnic background of the population (Weiss et al. 1995): e.g. 1.8% in the Hispano-American population (DeCosimo et al. 1987), 0.17% in Venezuela (Arevalo 1991), and less than 0.1% in France and Denmark (Jensen and Faber 1988; Sapin et al. 1989). So far there have been no reports of FDH in African or Asian subjects.

The most common albumin variant in FDH (type I FDH) has an increased affinity only for T_4. Type II FDH has an increased affinity fot T_4 and rT_3 and type III FDH an increased affinity for T_4, T_3 and rT_3; in type IV, T_3 and T_4 are sometimes affected (Bartalena 1990; Hennemann et al. 1979; Moses et al. 1982; Yabu et al. 1987). Recently it has been demonstrated that in FDH patients a missense mutation in position 218 (Arg-His) of the albumin gene results in the enhanced T_4 binding (Sunthornthepvarakul et al. 1994; Petersen et al. 1994).

Complete absence or polymorphism of albumin are rare conditions (Bartalena 1990) that have no effect on thyroid function tests, because of increased TBG and/or TTR concentrations in these subjects (Robbins 1973; Andreoli and Robbins 1962).

Table 9. Types of variant albumin in FDH: changes in binding affinity to thyroid hormones

	Binding to		
	T_4	T_3	rT_3
Type I	↑	Normal	Normal
Type II	↑	Normal	↑
Type III	↑	↑	↑
Type IV	(↑)	↑	Normal

To date, few cases of FDH with thyroid disorders have been reported: there was one patient with FDH and hypothyroidism secondary to Hashimoto's thyroiditis (YOUNG et al. 1987), two patients with FDH and thyrotoxicosis due to post-partum thyroiditis (LANGSTEGER et al. 1994a) and to subacute thyroiditis (CROXSON et al. 1985) respectively, and also two patients with FDH and hyperthyroid Graves' disease (YOUNG et al. 1987; JONES et al. 1987).

3.2 Acquired Albumin Variants

Acquired hyperthyroxinaemia can be also produced by mechanisms independent of changes in thyroid hormone-binding proteins, such as drugs, acute psychiatric disordes, generalized resistance to thyroid hormone and others (STOCKIGT 1993; REFETOFF 1992). For details and review see STOCKIGT (1993) and BARTALENA and ROBBINS (1992).

3.3 Thyroid Function Parameters

The practical relevance of FDH is the possibility of erroneous interpretation of thyroid function tests leading to inappropriate treatment modalities for thyrotoxicosis (EBER et al. 1991). Elevated serum TT_4 values and abnormally high analogue FT_4 (aFT4) values are highly suggestive of FDH. As would be expected, the two-step FT_4 and FT_4 values (FT_4-d) measured according to the method of STERLING and BRENNER (1966; STERLING and HEGEDUS 1962) by equilibrium dialysis are normal. More rarely, the serum rT_3 and, to some extent, the TT_3 concentrations are also significantly higher in family members affected by FDH. However, serum TSH concentrations (and, as already mentioned, free T_4 concentrations measured by equilibrium dialysis) are normal in all FDH subjects, confirming their clinical euthyroid state and additionally indicating an abnormality of thyroid hormone transport proteins in serum.

Autoimmune thyroid disease does not normally appear to be related to FDH (WEISS et al. 1995); nevertheless, a high prevalence of positive thyroid autoantibodies (TgAb, Mab, TPOAb) has been previously observed in Amish families by PAULS et al. (1993). Other tests of thyroid function (e.g. FT_3, TSH receptor autoantibodies, Tg, SHBG) are normal, compatible with the eumetabolic state of the affected subjects.

4 Transthyretin

Transthyretin (TTR), also called TBPA (T_4-binding prealbumin), a 55-kDa tetramer (REFETOFF 1979b) consisting of four identical subunits (FELDING and FEX 1982), is synthezised in the liver, pancreas islet cells and choroid plexus (MAYE et al. 1989; SCHREIBER et al. 1990; HERBERT et al. 1986). TTR only binds one T_4 molecule, because the first T_4 molecule eminently decreases the binding affinity of the second binding site; furthermore, one retinol-binding protein molecule will also be bound (BARTALENA 1990; CHENG et al. 1977; IRACE and EDELHOCH 1978; TRAGARDH et al. 1980; VAN JAARSVELD et al. 1973). Details of the physicochemical properties and binding characteristics are given in Tables 1–4.

Although the liver is the major producer of TTR in absolute terms, the epithelial cells of the choroid plexus contain at least 100 times more TTR mRNA per gram of tissue, thus demonstrating the important physiological role of TTR in the central nervous system (CNS) (SCHREIBER et al. 1990; HERBERT et al. 1986). T_4 penetrates the epithelial cells of the choroid plexus, binds to in situ synthesized TTR, and then enters the cerebrospinal fluid (CSF) as the TTR-T_4 complex. The distribution of T_4 to different regions of the CNS may play an important role during development (BARTALENA 1990; SCHREIBER et al. 1990).

4.1 Inherited TTR Variants

TTR-associated variations of thyroid hormone transport proteins (Tables 5, 6) appear to have an autosomal dominant inheritance pattern. Prealbumin-associated hyperthyroxinaemia (PAAH) was first described in 1982 by MOSES et al. About 18 TTR variants, with increased, reduced, or normal affinity for T_4, and characterized by different single amino acid substitutions, have been identified (BARTALENA and ROBBINS 1992; BARTALENA 1990; MOSES et al. 1990; LALLOZ et al. 1984). Patients with a similar condition which can be termed transthyretin-associated hyperthyroxinaemia (TTR-AH), in which TTR also has an increased affinity for rT_3 (Table 10) have also been described (LALLOZ et al. 1984).

Although this abnormality is apparently rare, it is likely to be more frequent than appears because even a fourfold increase in the affinity of TTR for T_4 is associated with normal serum T_4 concentrations (BARTALENA and ROBBINS 1992). Investigations of T_4 binding (REFETOFF et al. 1986; ROSEN et al. 1991) in TTR variants associated with familial amyloidotic polyneuropathy (FAP) or systemic amyloidosis have shown that the abnormal TTR is a major constituent of the amyloid fibril (BARTALENA 1990). These TTR variants have also a decreased affin-

Table 10. Types of inherited variants of TTR: changes in binding affinity to thyroid hormones

	T_4	T_3	rT_3
Type I	↑	Normal	Normal
Type II	↑	Normal	↑

Table 11. Acquired variants of TTR: changes in serum concentrations of TTR

Serum concentration of TTR	
Increased	Decreased
Endocrine pancreas tumours: insulinomas, glucagonomas Gut carcinoids	Nonthyroidal illness Trauma Alzheimer's disease
Drugs: androgens	Calorie deprivation Inflammatory stress
CNS disorders (CSF): Parkinson's disease, depression	Drugs: EMD 21388 Oestrogens

ity for T_4 because of an interaction of Thr^{109} with the hormone or with Ala^{108} and Leu^{110}, which are two components of the hydrophobic patch at the T_4 binding site (MOSES et al. 1990; REFETOFF et al. 1986; ROSEN et al. 1953).

4.2 Acquired TTR Variants

Acquired TTR-AH differs from inherited TTR variants, since serum TTR concentrations in the latter are normal; hyperthyroxinaemia in the inherited forms results from the increased T_4 affinity of TTR. The acquired variants of TTR (Table 11) are associated with drugs such as salicylates and penicillin (CAVALIERI and PITT-RIVES 1981; ROBBINS and RALL 1983). It can also be caused externally by nonthyroidal illness, malnutrition (BENVENGA et al. 1990; BARTALENA and ROBBINS 1992; INGENBLECK 1972), CNS disorders and endocrine pancreas tumors (BARTALENA and ROBBINS 1992; RAJATANAVIN et al. 1985). Two of these changes will be discussed now in more detail.

4.2.1 Central Nervous System

In patients with Alzheimer's disease (RIISOEN 1988), the TTR concentration in the CSF is inversely related to the degree of dementia. Patients with untreated endogenous depression have – possibly due to an association with increased TTR synthesis in the choroid plexus (JORGENSEN 1988) – increased levels of TTR in the CSF, which normalize as the depression lifts (JORGENSEN 1988). In Parkinson's disease a sustained increase in CSF TTR levels was seen after adrenal autotransplantation (ABRAM et al. 1990). However, these CNS disorders are not associated with changes in serum TTR or thyroid hormone concentrations.

4.2.2 Endocrine Tumours of the Pancreas

The high serum TTR concentration found in patients with insulinomas, glucagonomas and intestinal carcinoids is the result of synthesis and secretion of TTR by the tumour (JACOBSSON et al. 1989, 1990). The longstanding increase in serum TTR levels also leads to an increase in serum TT_4, with the typical pattern of euthyroid hyperthyroxinaemia (MAYE et al. 1989; RAJATANAVIN et al. 1985; JACOBSSON et al. 1989).

It should also be mentioned that EMD 21388, a synthetic flavonoid, selectively displaces T_4 from TTR (MENDEL et al. 1992; KÖHRLE et al. 1989; LUEPRASITSAKUL et al. 1990), resulting in a decreased T_4 fraction bound to TTR (MENDEL et al. 1992).

5 Methods of Separation of Thyroid Hormone-Binding Proteins

Various screening methods have been developed for the detection and evaluation of abnormal thyroid hormone-binding proteins (DOCTER et al. 1981; WAKONIG et al. 1987; STOCKIGT et al. 1986; LEOPOLD et al. 1987; WAWSCHINEK et al. 1987; ROBBINS and RALL 1952); some of them are mentioned in Table 12. Early attempts with paper electrophoresis failed, because of poor separation and artefacts due to the adsorption of albumin-bound T_4 on the filter paper (ROBBINS and RALL 1952). Better separation of albumin from TBG and TTR was achieved with reverse flow zone electrophoresis, introduced by PREMACHANDRA et al. (1967); but this technique is time-consuming and does not produce satisfactory separation. The agarose gel electrophoresis achieved by DOCTER et al. (1981) performed better separation, but had two major problems: cooling the slides in petroleum spirit, and cutting the thin gel for counting.

Table 12. Separation methods for thyroid hormone transport proteins

Paper electrophoresis
Reverse flow zone electrophoresis
Agarose gel electrophoresis
^{125}I-T_4 charcoal uptake/PEG precipitation
Tube cell agarose gel electrophoresis
Radial immune diffusion method
^{125}I-T_4/T_3 horizontal agarose gel electrophoresis

To avoid inappropriate treatment of patients, it was necessary to establish a rapid, accurate, simple, routinely available, highly reproducible and easy-to-perform method for determination of these proteins.

5.1 Horizontal Agarose Gel Low-Temperature Electrophoresis

Thyroxine binding to albumin, TTR and TBG was determined by agarose gel electrophoresis using a modified technique (WAKONIG et al. 1987) introduced by us, based on the agarose gel technique described by DOCTER et al. (1981). The modification allows in addition determination of peripheral T_3 and T_4 autoantibodies in one and the same procedure (WAKONIG et al. 1987).

Fresh or deep frozen serum (100 μl) is incubated with 5 μl radioactively labelled (7.4 Mbq/ml) ^{125}I-T_4 thyroxine solution (I.M. 141, Amersham, UK, containing 4 ng/μl T_4) and ^{125}I-T_3 triiodothyronine solution (I.M. 321, Amersham, UK, containing 4 ng/μl T_3) for 1 h at room temperature. To stain for albumin, the sera are mixed with 2.5 μl saturated aqueous bromophenol blue solution.

The serum sample (2.5 μl) is applied to a layer of agarose gel on a perfectly planar microscope slide. The agarose gel is prepared by dissolving 9 g agar purum (Behring, Marburg, Germany) in 1 l glycine acetate buffer solution (glycine 0.17 mol/l, acetic acid 0.13 mol/l, sodium hydroxide 0.14 mol/l, and sodium azide 3.1 mol/l). The buffer, with a pH of 8.6, also serves as a medium for the radiolabelled T_4/T_3 agarose low-temperature electrophoresis.

Separation is effected with a current of 250 mA over a period of 60–90 min in a vessel cooled to −13°C (Refrigerated Recirculator 486, Biorad, Austria). The gel is then cut into 25 strips of 2 mm width each, with a cutting device specially designed for that purpose. The individual gel strips are subjected to centrifugation in test tubes, which are then measured in a gamma counter. Evaluation and graphic display are computerized, using software specially developed for this application. The number of counts under each peak gives the binding of radioactively labelled T_4 or T_3 to TBG, albumin and TTR as a percentage of the total radioactivity (Table 13).

Either tube cell agarose gel electrophoresis (LEOPOLD et al. 1987) or the radial immune diffusion method (WAWSCHINEK et al. 1987) are best suited to cross-checking all the analyses.

Table 13. Normal distribution(%) of ^{125}I-T_4/T_3 in agarose gel electrophoresis

	Binding		Assay	
	T_4	T_3	cv % intra	cv % inter
TBG	70–92	81–94	1.1	2.9
Albumin	1–7	6–29	8.5	10.1
TTR	6–30	0–2	3.9	7.1

5.2 Scatchard Analysis

An additional Scatchard analysis (SCATCHARD 1949) should be carried out because electrophoretic methods cannot be used to calculate the affinity constant (K_a) of TBG, TTR and albumin. Maximum binding capacity (MBC) can be measured with agar gel electrophoresis (even in the presence of FDH albumin) by choosing a higher cold T_4 concentration to saturate the TBG or TTR, but this usually results in higher values.

6 Results of Thyroid Function Tests

When diagnosing thyroid hormone-binding variants, the selection of the methods used for free thyroid hormone estimation is the crucial point. Some assays, especially analogue methods, are very often affected by changes in the concentration or affinity of TBG, TTR or albumin, thus leading to artifactual and/or false high or even low results (BARTALENA and ROBBINS 1992; see BARTALENA et al. 1987 and EKINS 1990 for review).

An increase in serum total thyroid hormone concentrations is not the same thing as thyrotoxicosis, especially if the clinical picture is quite different. The "true" euthyroid status can readily – and indeed only – be established by measuring TSH and free thyroid hormone values (Table 14). The use of free thyroid hormone assays that have a good working performance and are also reliable when they suggest binding abnormalities is, therefore, one of the most decisive things.

To avoid spuriously high results, FT_4 and/or FT_3 have to be separated by equilibrium dialysis, ultrafiltration, column adsorption chromatography and immunoadsorption before radioimmunoassay (BARTALENA et al. 1987). The interaction of the labelled analogue with serum proteins and/or thyroid hormone autoantibodies gives inappropriately low values during pregnancy and in nonthyroid illness (because of the low-albumin condition). In FDH, TTR-AH, and in the presence of T_4/T_3 autoantibodies, spuriously high results will be given (BARTALENA et al. 1987).

Table 14. Thyroid function tests in individuals with thyroid hormone transport protein variants

	aFT_4	$2FT_4$	FT_4-d	TT_4	TBG	TT_3	rT_3	TSH
TBG-X	n	n	n	⇑	⇑	⇑	⇑	n
TBG-CD	n	n	n	⇓	⇓	⇓	⇓	n
FDH type I	⇑	n	n	⇑	n	n,⇑	n,⇑	n
TTR-AH type I	⇑	n	n	⇑	n	n	n,⇑	n

n, normal.

The coexistence of thyroid hormone transport protein variants with thyroid disorders (Table 7), such as Graves' disease or Hashimoto's thyroiditis, produces atypical thyroid function test abnormalities which can masquerade as thyroid hormone dysfunction (BARTALENA and ROBBINS 1992; REFETOFF 1989; NAKGAWA et al. 1967; HANSTED and MOLLER 1984; LANGSTEGER et al. 1994a; YOUNG et al. 1987; CROXSON et al. 1985; JONES et al. 1987). Thus, serum TT_4 and TT_3 values may be normal in hypothyroid patients; in hyperthyroid patients the differential diagnosis of increased serum T_4 and T_3 levels will become extremely difficult, because highly elevated serum TT_4 levels will be seen when giving a T_4 replacement or suppressive therapy (BARTALENA and ROBBINS 1992; LANGSTEGER et al. 1994b; YOUNG et al. 1987). Typical thyroid function tests results with inherited binding protein variants are shown in Table 15.

Combinations of binding protein abnormalities (Table 16), such as TBG deficiency with FDH (LANGSTEGER et al. 1994b), FDH in conjunction with TBG excess (YEO et al. 1987), FDH with enhanced TTR binding of T_4 (LALLOZ et al. 1987) and cases of a homozygous FDH syndrome (GERBER et al. 1988), are extremely rare, but produce further diagnostic difficulties (BARTALENA and ROBBINS 1992; REFETOFF 1989).

6.1 Disorders of TBG

As already mentioned, TBG, which carries more than 70% of T_4 and T_3, is the main serum protein responsible for substantial changes in thyroid hormone-binding

Table 15. Thyroid function tests in individuals with inherited thyroid hormone transport protein variants

	aFT_4 (9–28.3 pmol/l)	$2FT_4$ (8.8–28 pmol/l)	TT_4 (45–115 nmol/1)	TBG (15–30 mg/l)	TT3 (0.9–2.92 nmol/l)	TSH (0.3–4.0 mU/l)
FDH	>65	12.48	127	21.35	2.33	2.22
TBG-PD	22.28	13.76	28.7	11.2	1.05	0.96
FDH + TBG-PD	>65	17.20	113	<0.1	0.63	3.1
FDH	>65	16.78	133	29.25	2.04	2.72
FDH + PPT	>65	58.6	174	32.3	3.74	<0.01

PPT, post partum thyroiditis.

Table 16. Coexistence of inherited transport protein variations

FDH + TTR-AH
FDH + TBG-X
FDH + TBG-PD

capacity (ROBBINS and BARTALENA 1986). Increased TBG levels result in increased serum concentrations of total T_4 and total T_3. Decreased serum TBG concentrations, congenital or acquired, result in a reduction of TT_4 and TT_3 levels to the low-normal or even hypothyroid range (BARTALENA and ROBBINS 1992; FEINSTEIN et al. 1982), accompanied by normal analogue FT_4 and two-step FT_4 values and normal TSH (ROBBINS and BARTALENA 1986; REFETOFF 1979, 1979; BARTALENA 1990).

6.2 Disorders of Albumin

An increased affinity of albumin may show spuriously high TT_4 values, and sometimes - in different FDH albumin variants - elevated TT_3 and rT_3 levels (BARTALENA and ROBBINS 1992).

The analogue FT_4 assay results in markedly elevated values and can be used routinely, as in our laboratory, as a screening test for protein-binding anomalies, especially in FDH. In contrast, the two-step FT_4 assay measures the free T_4 concentration appropriately even in patients with FDH (RAJATANAVIN et al. 1982). Thus, FDH, suspected on the basis of markedly elevated analogue FT_4 and TT_4 values but normal serum TSH and two-step FT_4 values, is confirmed by $^{125}I-T_4/T_3$ agarose gel electrophoresis.

No changes of serum thyroid hormone levels are seen in the complete absence of albumin (analbuminaemia); this can readily be explained by a concomitant increase in serum TBG and/or TTR (BARTALENA and ROBBINS 1992; BARTALENA 1990).

6.3 Disorders of TTR

Elevated TTR levels (e.g. in endocrine tumours of the pancreas) may cause elevated TT_4 levels; no changes are seen in serum TT_3 concentrations. A decrease in the concentration or affinity of TTR (for T_4) may also affect thyroid hormone levels (LIND et al. 1990).

6.4 T_4/T_3 Autoantibodies

Depending on the separation method used, autoantibodies directed against T_3 and T_4 may cause changes in serum TT_4 and TT_3 values. Falsely high (double-antibody technique) or falsely low values (PEG precipitation or charcoal methods) will be seen when separating bound from free hormone by radioimmunoassay (BENVENGA et al. 1987).

6.5 TBG Deficiency with FDH

When FDH (type I) and TBG deficiency coexist, analogue FT_4 remains very high, two-step FT_4 is normal and due to the TBG deficiency the TT_4 values are normal (LANGSTEGER et al. 1994b).

Normal TT_4 concentrations despite TBG deficiency are consistent with the presence of dysalbuminaemia; when the variant albumin-like protein of FDH does not bind T_3, low serum TT_3 values, consistent with TBG deficiency, will not be masked. Serum rT_3 concentrations are not reduced, presumabley because an increased proportion is carried on the abnormal albumin-like protein.

The electrophoretic pattern of serum binding of $^{125}I\text{-}T_4$ may also be confusing, since increased binding of $^{125}I\text{-}T_4$ in the albumin and TTR zone occurs. The metabolic status of the subject can then only be surmised from the serum TSH level (LANGSTEGER et al. 1994b).

7 Results of Agarose Gel Electrophoresis

7.1 Normal Subjects

Figure 1 shows the normal distribution and the normal binding of T_4 and T_3 to TBG, TTR and albumin in a 24-year-old euthyroid subject without FDH. As already mentioned, the number of counts gives the binding of T_4 or T_3 to the three major transport proteins as a percentage of the total radioactivity.

7.2 Familial Dysalbuminaemic Hyperthyroxinaemia

In Fig. 2 the typical binding in FDH (type I) is shown: increased binding of T_4 to albumin and reduced binding of T_4 to TBG (T_4-binding shift from TBG to albumin). As expected, the T_3-binding curve does not have a pathological distribution and is therefore not shown.

7.3 Complete TBG Deficiency

Figure 3 shows the typical pattern of a subject with complete TBG deficiency: almost no binding of T_4 to TBG, slightly increased binding of T_4 to albumin and markedly enhanced binding of T_4 to the TTR zone (T_4-binding shift from TBG to albumin and TTR). The binding of T_3 to TBG, TTR and albumin is almost identical with the T_4-binding curve and is therefore not shown.

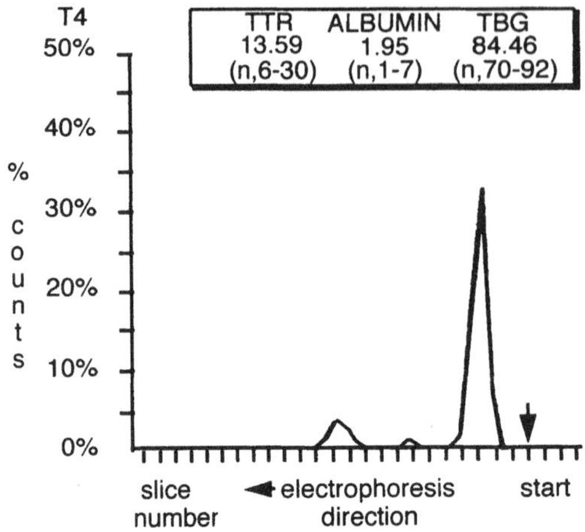

a

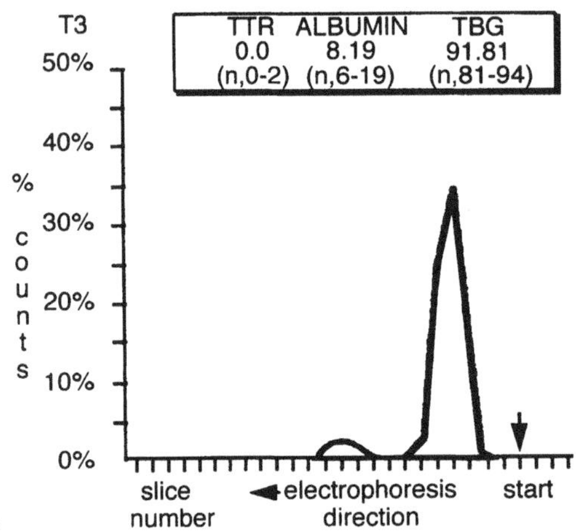

b

Fig. 1a,b. Normal distribution and binding of T_4 (**a**) and T_3 (**b**) to TBG, TTR, and albumin in a 24-year-old euthyroid subject

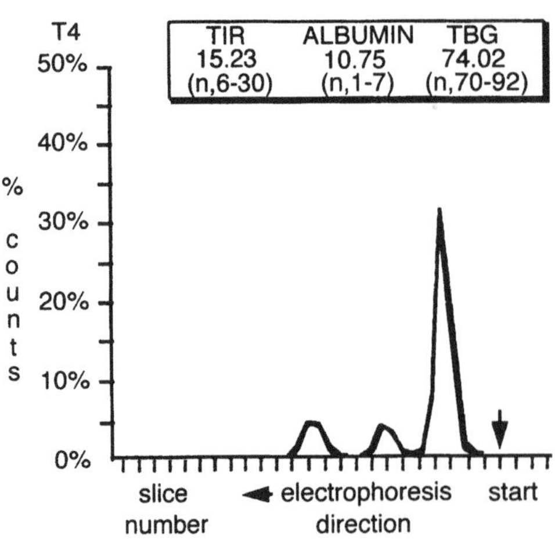

Fig. 2. Typical binding in FDH (type I)

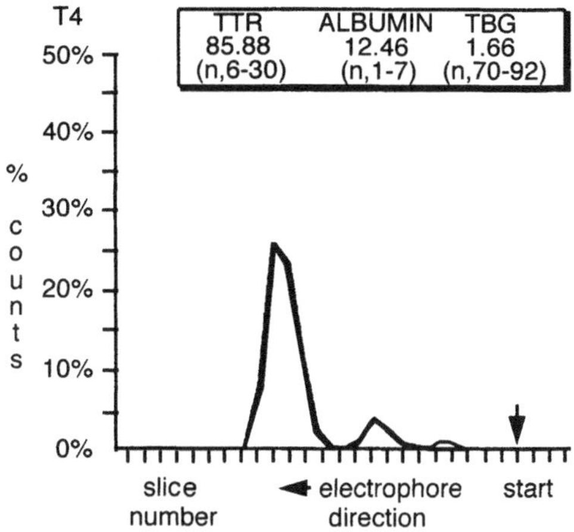

Fig. 3. Typical pattern of a subject with complete TBG deficiency

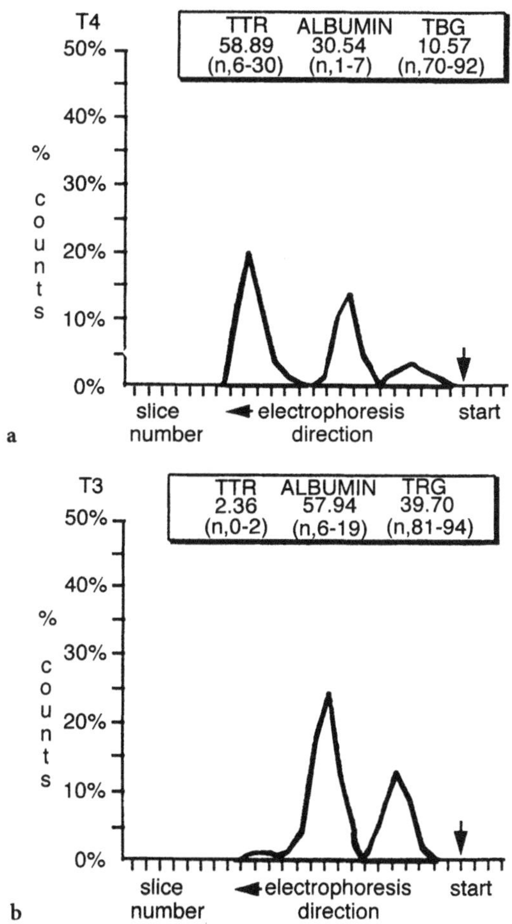

Fig. 4a,b. T_4 (**a**) and T_3 (**b**) binding in TBG deficiency with concomitant FDH (type I)

7.4 TBG Deficiency with Concomitant FDH (Type I)

T_4 binding (Fig. 4) in this combined anomaly is completely unreasonable: T_4 binding to TBG is decreased markedly (only about 15% of normal values), T_4 binding to albumin is almost 4.5-fold increased and T_4 binding to TTR doubles. The T_3 binding curve (Fig. 4b) shows markedly reduced T_3 binding to TBG and increased binding to albumin.

Evidence indicating a combined anomaly can be verified only in the following way: increasing quantities of TBG standards (e.g. 8.5, 40, 80 μl/ml) are added in vitro to the certain serum enriched with ^{125}I-T_4 in order to determine the shift of T_4 binding from albumin and TTR to TBG. As shown in Fig. 5a, after the in vitro addition of 80 μg TBG/ml serum (or about four times the normal concentration), normal T_4 binding to TTR – corresponding to the normal distribution of T_4 – can be observed. However, the elevated T_4 binding to albumin cannot be reduced, giving the typical pattern of FDH.

The binding of T_3 (Fig. 5b) shifts from albumin to TBG with increasing additions of TBG, ending when normal binding of T_3 to TBG is achieved; the binding of T_3 to albumin then corresponds to a normal distribution.

To cross-check these results, similar determinations with serum samples from a patient with pure TBG deficiency also reveal a shift of T_4 binding (Fig. 6a) from albumin and TTR to TBG; as expected, a normal distribution of T_4 binding and also of T_3 binding (Fig. 6b) amongst the binding proteins is shown.

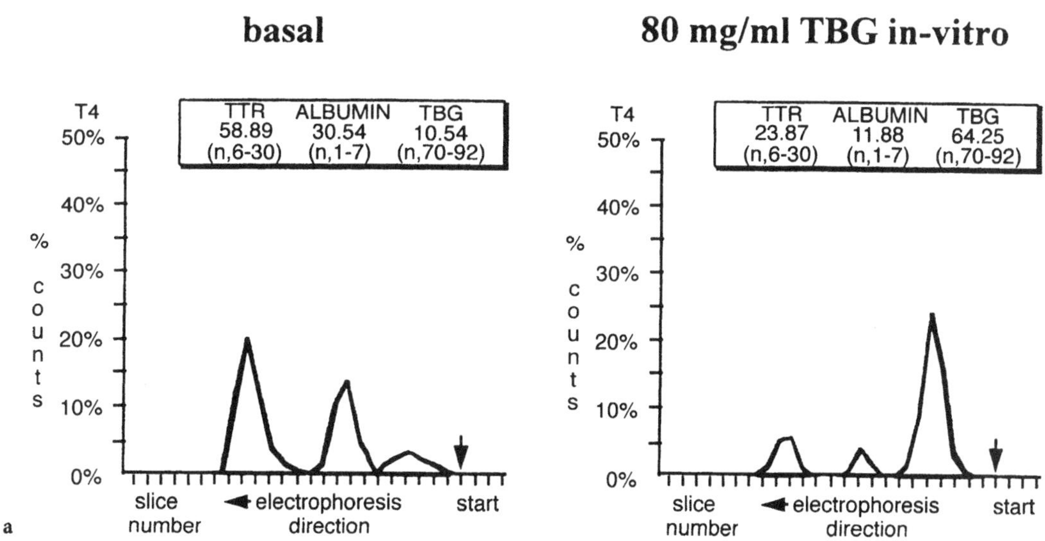

Fig. 5a,b. T_4 (a) and T_3 (b) binding in TBG deficiency with concomitant FDH (type I) before and after addition of 80 μg TBG/ml serum

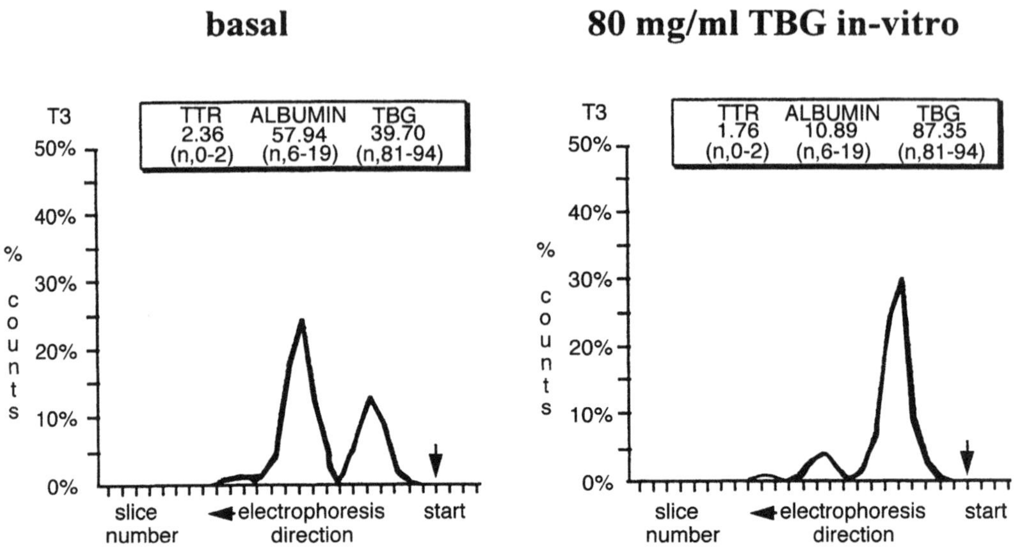

Fig. 5b

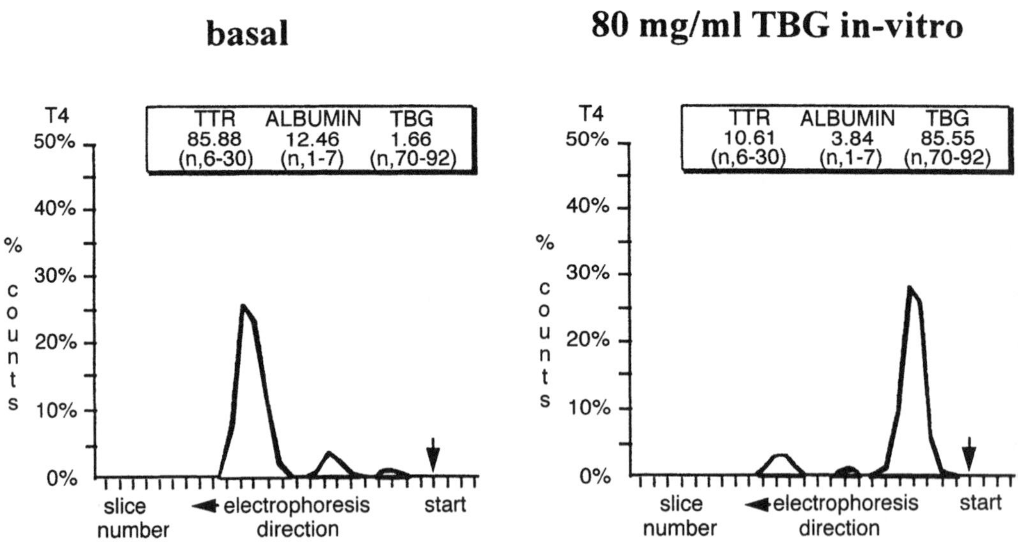

a

Fig. 6a,b. T_4 (**a**) and T_3 (**b**) binding in pure TBG deficiency

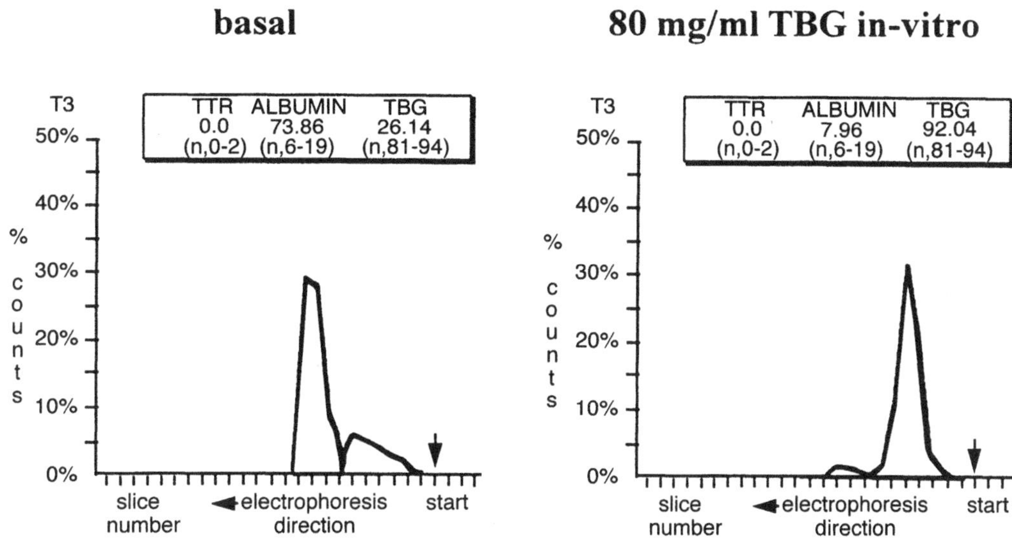

Fig. 6b

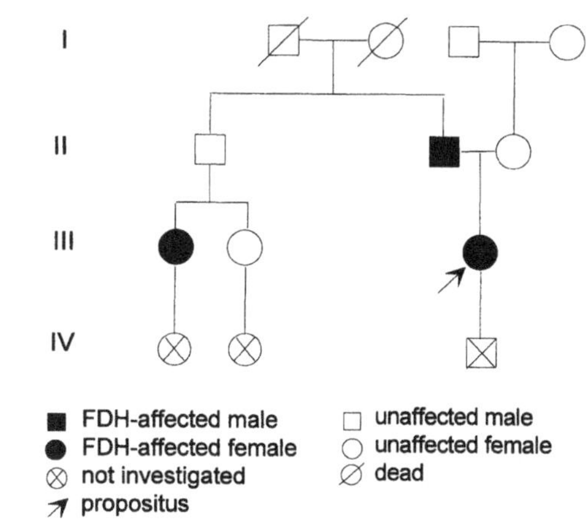

Fig. 7. Typical FDH family

8 Family Screening for Variant Binding Proteins

8.1 Familial Dysalbuminaemic Hyperthyroxaemia

Figure 7 shows a typical FDH family. Usually about 50% of family members are affected.

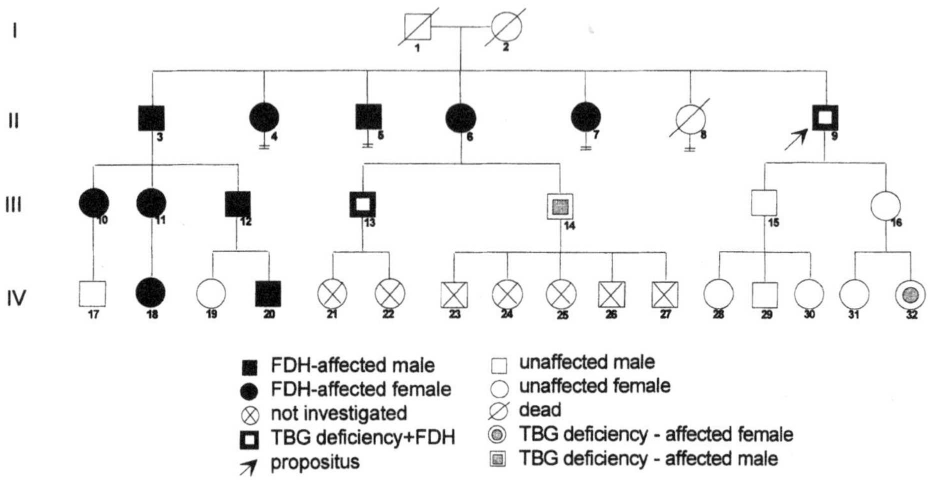

Fig. 8. Family tree of a family with a combined anomaly (TBG deficiency with FDH)

8.2 FDH and Partial TBG Deficiency

The family tree of a combined anomaly (TBG deficiency with FDH) is shown in Fig. 8. FDH was inherited from either the propositus' father or his mother, whereas the TBG deficiency was presumably transmitted through the mother. Failure to observe partial TBG deficiency in obligatory heterozygous subject 16 can be explained by the Lyon hypothesis (LYON 1962): that variable expression of the two X-chromosome alleles is characteristic of X-linked traits and is attributed to random, though uneven, X-chromosome inactivation in somatic cells.

9 Conclusion

Variations in the serum concentrations of TBG, TTR and albumin, either inherited or acquired, are quite common; most often TBG is involved, although changes in TTR and albumin are becoming more frequent.

The clinical impact of the interpretation and diagnosis of variations in thyroid hormone transport proteins is to protect patients from unnecessary, sometimes even contraindicated treatment. Two clinical studies (WYNNE et al. 1992; LANGSTEGER et al. 1993) have demonstrated that most patients with variant transport proteins were referred for thyroid testing because of incidentally detected "unusual" thyroid function test results. Although in most cases no palpable thyroid abnormalities were found, the interpretation of these unexpected thyroid function tests very often led to inappropriate treatment with surgery, ^{131}-I, antithyroid drugs alone or after surgery or ^{131}-I therapy, or T_4 replacement therapy.

Difficulties in the interpretation of thyroid function tests will, as already mentioned, still occur if changes in thyroid hormone transport proteins are seen in individuals who have thyroid disorders or in individuals who have two coexisting inherited transport protein defects.

References

Abram SR, Kruskal JB, Allen GS, Burns RS, Parker B, Tulipan N (1990) Alterations in prealbumin concentration after adrenal autotransplantation for Parkinson's disease. Exp Neurol 108: 130–135

Abuid J, Larsen PR (1974) Triiodothyronine and thyroxine in hyperthyroidism: comparison of the acute changes during therapy with antihyroid agents. J Clin Invest 54: 201–207

Ain KB, Mori Y, Refetoff S (1987) Reduced clearance rate of thyroxine-binding globulin (TBG) with increased sialylation: a mechanism for estrogen-induced elevation of serum TBG concentration. J Clin Endocrinol Metab 65: 689–696

Ain KB, Refetoff S (1988) Relationship of oligosaccharide modification to the cause of serum thyroxine-binding globulin excess. J Clin Endocrinol Metab 66: 1037–1043

Alexopoulos A, Hutchinson W, Bari A, Keating JJ, Johnson PJ, Williams R (1988) Hyperthyroxinaemia in hepatocellular carcinoma: relation to thyroid binding globulin in the clinical and preclinical stages of the disease. Br J Cancer 57: 313–317

Amino N, Yabu Y, Miki T et al (1981) Serum ratio of triiodothyronine to thyroxine, and thyroxine-binding globulin and calcitonin concentrations in Graves' disease and destruction-induced thyrotoxicosis. J Clin Endocrinol Metab 53: 113–116

Andreoli M, Robbins J (1962) Serum proteins and thyroxine protein interactions in early human fetuses. J Clin Invest 41: 1070–1077

Arevalo G (1991) Prevalence of familial dysalbuminemic hyperthyoxinemia in serum samples received for thyroid testing. Clin Chem 37: 1430–1431

Barlow JW, Csicsmann JM, Meinhold H, Lim CF, Stockigt JR (1986) Familial dysalbuminaemic hyperthyroxinemia: study of albumin binding and implications for hormone action. Clin Endocrinol (Oxf) 24: 39–47

Bartalena L (1990) Recent achievements in studies on thyroid hormone-binding proteins. Endocr Rev 1: 47–63

Bartalena L, Robbins J (1984) Effect of tunicamycin and monensin on secretion of thyroxine-binding globulin by cultured human hepatoma (Hep G2) cells. J Biol Chem 259: 13610–13614

Bartalena L, Robbins J (1992) Variations in thyroid hormone transport proteins and their clinical implications. Thyroid 3: 237–245

Bartalena L, Grimaldi S, Fleischmann K, Robbins J (1986a) Biosynthesis of a novel thyroxine-binding protein (27 K protein) in human hepatoma (Hep G2) cells. Endocrinology 118: 2370–2377

Bartalena L, Grimaldi S, Robbins J (1986b) Human hepatoma (Hep G2) cells secrete a novel T_4-binding protein (27 K protein). In: Medeiors-Neto G, Gaitan E (eds) Frontiers in thyroidology. Plenum, New York, pp 477–512

Bartalena L, Martino E, Antonelli A, Pacchiarotti A, Robbins J, Pinchera A (1986c) Effect of the antileukemic agent L-asparaginase on thyroxine-binding globulin and albumin synthesis in cultured human hepatoma (Hep G2) cells. Endocrinology 119: 1185–1188

Bartalena L, Mariotti S, Pinchera A (1987) Radioimmunoassay of thyroid hormones. In: Patrono C, Peskar BA (eds) Handbook of experimental pharmacology, vol 82. Springer, Berlin Heidelberg New York, pp 401–431

Benvenga S (1989) The 27-kilodalton thyroxine (T_4)-binding protein is human apolipoprotein A-I: identification of a 68-kilodalton high density lipoprotein that binds T_4. Endocrinology 124: 1265–1269

Benvenga S, Robbins J (1987) Enhancement of thyroxine entry into low density lipoprotein (LDL) receptor-competent fibroblasts by LDL: an additional mode of entry of thyroxine into cells. Endocrinology 126: 933–941

Benvenga S, Trimarchi F, Robbins J (1987) Circulating thyroid hormone autoantibodies. J Endocrinol Invest 10: 606–619

Benvenga S, Gregg RE, Robbins J (1988) Binding of thyroid hormones to human plasma lipoproteins. J Clin Endocrinol Metab 67: 6–16

Benvenga S, Cahnmann HJ, Gregg RE, Robbins J (1989) Characterization of the binding of thyroxine to high density lipoproteins and apolipoproteins A-I. J Clin Endocrinol Metab 68: 1067–1072

Benvenga S, Cahnmann HJ, Robbins J (1990) Localization of the thyroxine binding sites in apolipoprotein B-100 of human low density lipoproteins. Endocrinology 127: 2241–2246

Bertenshaw R, Takeda K, Refetoff S (1991) Sequencing of the variant throxine-binding globulin (TBG)-Quebec reveals two nucleotide substitutions. Am J Hum Genet 48: 741–744

Bianchi R, Iervasi G, Pilo A, Vitek F, Ferdeghini M, Cazzuola F, Giraudi G (1987) Role of serum carrier proteins in the peripheral metabolism and tissue distribution of thyroid hormones in familial dysalbuminemic hyperthyroxinemia and congenital elevation of thyroxine binding globulin. J Clin Invest 80: 522–534

Brown SK, Bellisario R (1986) Measurement of thyroxine-binding globulin (TBG) levels from dried blood spot specimens: detection of TBG deficiency and TBG excess in infants. In: Carter TP, Wiley AM (eds) Genetic disease: screening and management. Liss, New York, pp 373–384

Burr WA, Ramsden DB, Hoffenberg R (1980) Hereditary abnormalities of thyroxine-binding globulin concentration: a study of 19 kindreds with inherited increase or decrease of thyroxine-binding globulin. Q J Med 49: 295–313

Cavalieri RR, McMahon FA, Castle JN (1975) Preparation of ^{125}I-labeled human thyroxine-binding alpha globulin and its turnover in normal and hypothyroid subjects. J Clin Invest 56: 79–84

Cavalieri RR, Pitt-Rivers R (1981) The effects of drugs on the distribution and metabolism of thyroid hormones. Pharmacol Rev 33: 55–80

Chan V, Besser GM, Landon J (1972) Effects of oestrogen on urinary thyroxine excretion. Br Med J 4: 699–703

Cheng SY, Pages RA, Saroff HA, Edelhoch H, Robbins J (1977) Analysis of thyroid hormone binding to human serum prealbumin by 8-anilinonaphthalene sulfonate fluorescence. Biochemistry 16: 3707–3712

Copping S, Byfield PGH (1988) Thyroxine-binding globulin deficiency re-examined. Clin Endocrinol (Oxf) 28: 45–51

Croxson MS, Palmer BN, Holdaway IM, Frengley PA, Evans MC (1985) Detection of familial dysalbuminaemic hyperthyroxinaemia. Br Med J 290: 1099–1102

Daiger SP, Rummel DP, Wang L, Cavalli-Sforza LL (1981) Detection of genetic variation with radioactive ligands. IV. X-linked, polymorphic genetic variation of thyroxin-binding globulin (TBG). Am J Hum Genet 33: 640–648

Daiger SP, Wildin RS (1981) Human thyroxine-binding globulin (TBG): heterogeneity within individuals and among individuals demonstrated by isoelectric focusing. Biochem Genet 19: 673–685

DeCosimo DR, Fang SL, Braverman LE (1987) Prevalence of familial dysalbuminemic hyperthyroxinemia in Hispanics. Ann Intern Med 107: 780–781

Dick M, Watson F (1981) A possible variant of thyroxine-binding globulin in Australian aborigines. Clin Chim Acta 116: 361–367

Divino CM, Schussler GC (1989) Transthyretin receptors on human astrocytoma cells. J Clin Endocrinol Metab 71: 1265–1268

Divino CM, Schussler GC (1990) Studies on the nature of iodothyronine binding in familial dysalbuminemic hyperthyroxinemia. J Clin Endocrinol Metab 71: 98–104

Docter R, Bos G, Krenning EP, Fekkes D, Visser TJ, Hennemann G (1981) Inherited thyroxine excess: a serum abnormality due to an increased affinity for modified albumin. Clin Endocrinol (Oxf) 15: 363–371

Docter R, Bos G, Krenning EP, Hennemann G (1984) Specific thyroxine binding albumine is a constituent of normal human serum. Lancet 1: 50

Eber O, Langsteger W, Florian W, Schubert B, Lind P, Klima G, Wawschinek O (1991) Evaluation of thyroid function in patients with protein binding anomalies. Acta Med Austriaca 1: 11–18

Ekins RP (1990) Measurement of free hormones in blood. Endocr Rev 11: 5–46
Ekins RP, Sinha A, Ballabio M et al (1989) Role of the maternal carrier proteins in the supply of thyroid hormones to the fetoplacental unit: evidence of a fetoplacental requirement for thyroxine. In: Delange F, Fisher DA, Glinoer D (eds) Research in congenital hypothyroidism. Plenum, New York, pp 45–60
Feinstein EL, Kaptein EM, Nicoloff JT, Massry SG (1988) Thyroid function in patients with nephrotic syndrome and normal renal function. Am J Nephrol 2: 70–76
Felding P, Fex G (1982) Cellular origin of prealbumin in the rat. Biochim Biophys Acta 716: 446
Flink IL, Bailey TJ, Gustafson TA, Markham BE, Morkin E (1986) Complete amino acid sequence of human thyroxine-binding globulin deduced from cloned DNA: close homology to the serine antiproteases. Proc Natl Acad Sci USA 83: 7708–7712
Gärtner R, Henze R, Horn K, Pickardt CR, Scriba PC (1981) Thyroxine-binding globulin: investigation of microheterogeneity. J Clin Endocrinol Metab 52: 657–664
Gerber H, Dekalbermatten N, König MP (1988) Genetic and critical challenges of familial dysalbuminemic hyperthyroxinemia (FDH). Ann Endocrinol (Paris) 49: 244(A)
Gershengorn MC, Cheng SY, Lippoldt RE, Lord RB, Robbins J (1977) Characterization of human thyroxine-binding globulin. Evidence for a single polypeptide chain. J Biol Chem 252: 8713–8723
Gerstner JB, Kaplan RH (1976) Hyperthyroidism with normal concentration of total serum thyroxine and triiodothyronine. J Clin Endocrinol Metab 42: 64–69
Glinoer D, Gershengorn MC, Dubois A, Robbins J (1977) Stimulation of thyroxine-binding globulin synthesis by isolated Rhesus monkey hepatocytes after in vivo fl-estradiol administration. Endocrinology 100: 807–813
Gordon AH, Gross J, O'Connor D, Pitt-Rivers R (1962) Nature of the circulating thyroid hormone-plasma protein complex. Nature 169: 19–20
Griffiths KD, Virdi NK, Rayner PHW, Green A (1985) Neonatal screening for congenital hypothyroidism by measurement of plasma thyroxine and thyroid stimulating hormone concentrations. Br Med J 291: 117–120
Grimaldi S, Robbins Z (1982) Effect of thyroxine on molecular properties of native and dausylated thyroxine-binding globulin. Eudocrinol Exp (Bratish) 16: 273–276
Grimaldi S, Edelhoch H, Robbins J (1982) Effects of thyroxine binding on the stability, conformation, and fluorescence porperties of thyroxine-binding globulin. Biochemistry 21: 145–149
Grimaldi S, Bartalena L, Ramacciotti C, Robbins J (1983) Polymorphism of human thyroxine-binding globulin. J Clin Endocrinol Metab 57: 1186–1192
Grimaldi S, Bartalena L, Carlini F, Robbins J (1986) Purification and partial characterization of a novel thyroxine-binding protein (27 K protein) from human plasma. Endocrinology 118: 2362–2368
Hammond GL, Smith CL, Goping IS, Underhill DA, Harley MJ, Reventos J, Musto NA, Gunsalus GL, Bardin CW (1987) Primary structure of human corticosteroid binding globulin, deduced from hepatic and pulmonary cDNAs, exhibits homology with serine protease inhibitors. Proc Natl Acad Sci USA 84: 5153–5157
Hansted LC, Moller A (1984) Congenital deficiency of thyroxin-binding globulin (TBG). Ugeskr Laeger 146: 4022–4024
Hashizume K, Sakurai A, Miyamoto T, Yamauchi K, Nishii Y (1986) Effect of thyroxine-binding globulin (TBG) on thyroxine (T_4) uptake by human peripheral mononuclear cells: evidence of TBG dependent uptake of T_4. Endocrinol Jpn 33: 665–669
Hennemann G, Docter R (1990) Plasma transport proteins and their role in tissue delivery of thyroid hormone. In: Greer MA (ed) The thyroid gland. Raven, New York, pp 221–231
Hennemann G, Docter R, Krenning EP, Bos G, Otten M, Visser TJ (1979) Raised total thyroxine and free thyroxine index but normal free thyroxine: a serum abnormality due to inherited increased affinity of iodothyronine for serum binding protein. Lancet 1: 639–642
Herbert J, Wilcox JN, Pham KTC, Fremeau RT, Zeviani M, Dwork A, Soprano DR, Makover A, Goodmann-Dewitt S, Zimmermann EA, Roberts JL, Schon EA (1986) Transthyretin: a choroid plexus-specific transport protein in human brain. Neurology 36: 900–907
Hochman G (1981) Human thyroxine binding globulin. Rev Physiol Biochem Pharmacol 81: 46–85

Horwitz DL, Refetoff S (1977) Graves' disease associated with familial deficiency of thyroxine-binding globulin. J Clin Endocrinol Metab 44: 242
Huang MJ, Liaw YF (1990) Thyroxine-binding globulin in patients with chronic hepatitis B virus infection: different implications in hepatitis and hepatocellular carcinoma. Am J Gastroenterol 85: 281–284
Inada M, Kasagi K, Kurata S et al (1975) Estimation of thyroxine and triiodothyronine distribution and of the conversion rate of thyroxine to triiodothyronine in man. J Clin Invest 55: 1337–1348
Ingbar SH (1961) Clinical and physiological observations in a patient with an idiopathic decrease in the thyroxine-binding globulin of plasma. J Clin Invest 40: 2053–2063
Ingenbleck Y (1972) Measurement of prealbumin as index of protein calorie malnutrition. Lancet 2: 106–109
Irace G, Edelhoch H (1978) Thyroxine-induced conformational changes in prealbumin. Biochemistry 17: 5729–5733
Ishizuki Y, Satoh S, Hirata S (1981) Hyperthyroidism associated with TBG deficiency. Saishin Igaku 36: 1026–1031
Jacobsson B, Caristrom A, Collins VP, Cornelius L (1989) Transthyretin in endocrine pancreatic tumors. Am J Pathol 134: 465–471
Jacobsson B, Caristrom A, Plotz A, Collins VP (1990) Transthyretin messenger ribonucleic acid expression in the pancreas and in endocrine tumors of the pancreas and gut. J Clin Endocrinol Metab 71: 875–880
Janssen OE, Bertenshaw R, Takeda K, Weiss R, Refetoff S (1992) Molecular basis of inherited thyroxine-binding globulin defects. Trends Endocrinol Metab 3: 49–53
Janssen OE, Takeda K, Refetoff S (1991) Sequence of the variant thyroxine-binding globulin (TBG) in a Montreal family with partial TBG deficiency. Hum Genet 87: 119–122
Jenkins MB, Steffes MW (1987) Congenital thyroxine binding globulin deficiency: incidence and inheritance. Hum Genet 77: 80–85
Jensen IW, Faber J, Grunnet N (1990) Familial occurrence of dysalbuminemic hyperthyroxinemia, lipomatosis and ankylosing spondylitis. Scand J Rheumatol 19: 303–305
Jensen IW, Faber J (1988) Familial dysalbuminaemic hyperthroxinaemia: a review. J R Soc Med 81: 34–37
Jones A, Hopton MR, Gurling KJ, Harrop JS (1987) Iatrogenic hypothyroidism and postpartum hyperthyroidism in familial dysalbuminaemic hyperthyroxinaemia. Br Med J 294: 286
Jorgensen OS (1988) Neural cell adhesion molecule (NCAM) and prealbumin in cerebrospinal fluid from depressed patients. Acta Psychiatr Scand 345: 29–37
Kamboh MI, Kirwood C (1984) Genetic polymorphism of thyroxine-binding globulin (TBG) in the Pacific area. Am J Hum Genet 36: 646–654
Kamikubo K, Kojima N, Yamakita N, Miura K (1985) A case of total thyroxine-binding globulin deficiency with Graves' disease: fluctuations of plasma triiodothyronine/thyroxine ratio. Jpn J Med 25: 186–190
Köhrle J, Fang SL, Yang Y, Irmscher K, Hesch RD, Pino S, Alex S, Braverman LE (1989) Rapid effects of the flavonoid EMD 21388 on serum thyroid hormone binding and thyrotropin regulation in the rat. Endocrinology 125: 532–537
Lalloz MR, Byfield PGH, Himsworth RL (1983) Hyperthyroxinemia: abnormal binding of T_4 by an inherited albumin variant. Clin Endocrinol (Oxf) 18: 11–24
Lalloz MRA, Byfield PGH, Goel KM, Loudon MM, Thomson JA, Himsworth RL (1987) Hyperthyroxinemia due to the coexistence of two raised affinity thyroxine-binding proteins (albumin and prealbumin) in one family. J Clin Endocrinol Metab 64: 346–352
Lalloz MRA, Byfield PGH, Himsworth RL (1986) A new and distinctive albumin variant with increased affinities for both triiodothyronines and causing hyperthyroxinemia: studies of albumin binding and implications for hormone action. Clin Endocrinol (Oxf) 24: 39–47
Lalloz MRA, Byfield PGH, Himsworth RL (1984) A prealbumin variant with an increased affinity for T_4 and reverse-T_3. Clin Endocrinol (Oxf) 21: 331–338
Lambert M, Zech F, DeNayer P, Jamez J, Vandercam B (1990) Elevation of serum thyroxine-binding globulin (but not of cortisol-binding globulin and sex hormone-binding globulin)

associated with the progression of human immunodeficiency virus infection. Am J Med 89: 748–751

Langsteger W, Költringer P, Semlitsch G, Meister E, Buchinger W, Eber O (1993) Evaluation and results of family screening in 126 FDH patients. Thyroid 3(S): T8(A)

Langsteger W, Semlitsch G, Költringer P, Meister E, Eber O (1994a) Post partum thyroiditis and familial dysalbumineic hyperthyroxinemia. J Clin Endocrinol Metab 78: 58–62

Langsteger W, Stockigt JR, Docter R, Költringer P, Lorenz O, Eber O (1994b) Familial dysalbuminaemic hyperthyroxinaemia and inherited partial TBG deficiency: first report. Clin Endocrinol (Oxf) 40: 751–758

Lao TT, Chin RKH, Panesar RS, Lam YM (1989) Birth weight and thyroxine-binding globulin in pre-eclampsia. Gynecol Obstet Invest 28: 8–10

Larsen PR (1972) Triiodothyronine: review of recent studies of its physiology and pathophysiology in man. Metabolism 21: 1073–1011

Leahy BC, Laing I, Davis D, Walton L (1984) High serum thyroxine-binding globulin – an important cause of hyperthyroxinaemia. Postgrad Med J 60: 324

Lee WNP, Golden MP, Van Herle AJ, Lippe BM, Kaplan SA (1979) Inherited abnormal thyroid hormone-binding protein causing selective increase of total serum thyroxine. J Clin Endocrinol Metab 49: 292–299

Leopold B, Wawschinek O, Lind P, Eber O (1987) Radioelectrophoresis for determination of thyroid hormone binding abnormalities in human serum. J Clin Chem Clin Biochem 25: 431–435

Li P, Janssen OE, Takeda K, Bertenshaw RH, Refetoff S (1991) Complete thyroxine-binding globulin (TBG) deficiency caused by a single nucleotide deletion in the TBG gene. Metabolism 41: 1231–1234

Lind P, Langsteger W, Költringer P, Wakonig P, Eber B, Mokry M, Beham A, Eber O (1990) Transient prealbumin-associated hyperthyroxinemia in TSH-producing pituitary adenoma. Nucl Med 29: 40–43

LoPresti JS, Fried JC, Spencer CA, Nicoloff JT (1989) Unique alterations of thyroid hormone indices in the acquired immunodeficiency syndrome (AIDS). Ann Intern Med 110: 970–975

Lueprasitsakul WS, Alex S, Fang SL, Pino S, Irmscher K, Köhrle J, Braverman LE (1990) Flavonoid administration immediately displaces thyroxine (T_4) from serum transthyretin, increases serum free T_4 and decreases serum thyrotropin in the rat. Endocrinology 126: 2890–2895

Lyon ICT (1983) Screening for hypothyroidism: the New Zealand experience. In: Naruse H, Irie M (eds) Neonatal screening international congress. Excerpta Medica, New York, pp 111–112

Lyon MR (1962) Sex chromatin and gene action in the mammalian X-chromosome. Am J Hum Genet 14: 135–140

Maye P, Bisetti A, Docter R, Gaillard R, Griessen M, Pelte MF (1989) Hyperprealbuminemia, euthyroid hyperthyroxinemia, Zollinger-Ellison-like syndrome and hypercorticism in a pancreatic endocrine tumour. Acta Endocrinol (Copenh) 120: 87–91

Mendel CM, Cavalieri RR (1984) Thyroxine distribution and metabolism in familial dysalbuminemic hyperthyroxinemia. J Clin Endocrinol Metab 59: 499–504

Mendel CM, Weisinger RA, Jones AL, Cavalieri RR (1987) Thyroid hormone-binding proteins in plasma facilitate uniform distribution of thyroxine within tissues: a perfused rat liver study. Endocrinology 120: 1742–1749

Mendel CM, Cavalieri RR, Köhrle J (1992) Thyroxine (T_4) transport and distribution in rats treated with EMD 21388, a synthetic flavonoid that displaces T_4 from transthyretin. Endocrinology 130: 1525–1532

Moloshok RE, Hsu LYF, Seal US, Hirschhorn K (1969) Partial thyroxine-binding globulin deficiency in a family. Pediatrics 44: 518

Mori Y, Refetoff S, Flink IL, Charbonneau M, Murata Y, Seo H, Horkin E, Dussault JH (1988) Detection of thyroxine-binding globulin (TBG) gene in six unrelated familes with complete TBG deficiency. J Clin Endocrinol Metab 67: 727–731

Mori Y, Takeda K, Charbonneau M, Refetoff S (1990) Replacement of Leu227 by Pro in thyroxine-binding globulin (TBG) is associated with complete TBG deficiency in three of eight familes with this inherited defect. J Clin Endocrinol Metab 70: 804–809

Moses AC, Lawlor J, Haddow J, Jackson IMD (1982) Familial euthyroid hyperthyroxinemia resulting from increased thyroxine binding to thyroxine-binding prealbumin. N Engl J Med 306: 966–969

Moses C, Rosen HN, Moller DE, Tsuzaki S, Haddow JE, Lawlor J, Liepniecks JJ, Nichols WC, Benson MD (1990) A point mutation in transthyretin increases affinity for thyroxine and produces euthyroid hyperthroxinemia. J Clin Invest 86: 2025–2033

Murata Y, Refetoff S, Sarne DH, Dick M, Watson F (1985) Variant thyroxine binding globulin in serum of Australian aborigines: its physical, chemical and biological properties. J Endocrinol Invest 8: 225–232

Murata Y, Sarne DH, Horwitz AL, Lecocq R, Aden DP, Knowles BB, Refetoff S (1985) Characterization of thyroxine-binding globulin secreted by a human hepatoma cell line. J Clin Endocrinol Metab 60: 472–478

Murata Y, Takamatsu J, Refetoff S (1986) Inherited abnormality of thyroxine-binding globulin with no demonstrable thyroxine-binding activity and high serum levels of denatured thyroxine-binding globulin. N Engl J Med 314: 694–699

Nakagawa M, Kinoshita Y, Yumoto Y (1967) A family of thyroxine-binding globulin deficiency. Folia Endocrinol Jpn 43: 248–251

Nikolai TF, Seal US (1966) X-chromosome linked familial decrease in thyroxine-binding globulin deficiency. J Clin Endocrinol Metab 25: 835–841

Oppenheimer JH (1968) Role of plasma proteins in the binding, distribution and metabolism of the thyroid hormones. N Engl J Med 278: 1153–1162

Pauls DL, Zakarija M, McKenzie M, Egeland JA (1993) Complex segregation analysis of antibodies to thyroid peroxidase in old order Amish families. Am J Med Genet 47: 375–379

Pemberton PA, Stein PE, Pepys MB, Potter JM, Carell RW (1988) Hormone binding globulins undergo serpin conformational change in inflammation. Nature 336: 257–267

Penhaligon J, Wellby ML (1982) Elevated serum thyroxine-binding globulin by X-chromosome transmission. Acta Endocrinol (Copenh) 99: 393–396

Peters T (1975) Serum albumin. In: Putnam FW (ed) The plasma proteins. Academic, New York, pp 131–181

Petersen CE, Scottolini AG, Cody LR, Mandel M, Reimer N, Bhagavan NV (1994) A point mutation in the human serum albumin gene results in familial dysalbuminaemic hyperthyroxinaemia. J Med Genet 31: 355–359

Premachandra BN, Blumenthal HT (1967) Abnormal binding of thyroid hormone in sera from patients with Hashimoto's disease. J Clin Endocrinol 27: 931–936

Rajatanavin R, Fournier L, DeCosimo D, Abreau CBS, Braverman LE (1982) Elevated serum free thyroxine by thyroxine analog radioimmunoassays in euthyroid patients with familial dysalbuminemic hyperthyroxinemia. Ann Intern Med 97: 865–866

Rajatanavin R, Liberman C, Lawrence GD, D'Arcangues CM, Young RA, Emerson C (1985) Euthyroid hyperthyroxinemia and thyroxine-binding prealbumin excess in islet cell carcinoma. J Clin Endocrinol Metab 61: 17–21

Refetoff S (1979a) Thyroid function tests. In: DeGroot LJ (ed) Endocrinology, vol 1. Grune and Stratton, New York, pp 387–428

Refetoff S (1979b) Thyroid hormone transport. In: DeGroot LJ (ed) Endocrinology, vol 1. Grune and Stratton, New York, pp 347–356

Refetoff S (1989) Inherited throxine-binding globulin (TBG) abnormalities in man. Endocr Rev 3: 275–293

Refetoff S (1992) Clinical and genetic aspects of resistnce to thyroid hormone. Endocrinologist 4: 261–271

Refetoff S, Larsen PR (1989) Transport, cellular uptake and metabolism of thyroid hormone. In: DeGroot LJ (ed) Endocrinology, 2nd edn. Saunders, Philadelphia, pp 541–561

Refetoff S, Murata Y (1985) X-chromosome-linked inheritance of the variant thyroxine-binding globulin in Australian aborigines. J Clin Endocrinol Metab 60: 356–360

Refetoff S, Selenkow HA (1968) Familial thyroxine-binding globulin deficiency in a patient with Turner's syndrome (XO): genetic study of a kindred. N Engl J Med 278: 1081–1087

Refetoff S, Robin NI, Alper CA (1972) Study of four new kindreds with inherited thyroxine-binding globulin abnormalities: possible mutations of a single gene locus. J Clin Invest 51: 848–867

Refetoff S, Fang VS, Marshall JS (1975) Studies on human thtroxine-binding globulin (TBG). IX. Some physical, chemical and biological properties of radioiodinated TBG and partially desialylated TBG (STBG). J Clin Invest 56: 177–187

Refetoff S, Fang VS, Marshall JS, Robin NI (1976) Metabolism of thyroxine-binding globulin (TBG) in man: abnormal rate of synthesis in inherited TBG deficiency and excess. J Clin Invest 57: 485–495

Refetoff S, Murata Y, Vassart G, Chandramouli V, Marshall JS (1984) Radioimmunoassays specific for the tertiary and primary structures of thyroxine-binding globulin (TBG): measurement of denatured TBG in serum. J Clin Endocrinol Metab 59: 269–277

Refetoff S, Dwulet FE, Benson MD (1986) Reduced affinity for thyroxine in two of three structural thyroxine-binding prealbumin variants associated with familial amyloidotic polyneuropathy. J Clin Endocrinol Metab 63: 1432–1437

Robbins J (1973) Inherited variations in thyroxine transport. Mt Sinai J Med 40: 511–519

Robbins J (1991) Thyroid hormone transport proteins and the physiology of hormone binding. In: Braverman LE, Utiger RD (eds) Werner's and Ingbar's the thyroid – a fundamental and clinical text. Lippincott, Philadelphia, pp 111–124

Robbins J, Bartalena L (1986) Plasma trasport of thyroid hormones. In: Hennemann G (ed) Thyroid hormone metabolism. Dekker, New York, pp 3–38

Robbins J, Rall JE (1952) Zone electrophoresis on filter paper of serum I-131 after radioiodine administration. Proc Soc Exp Biol Med 81: 530–536

Robbins J, Rall JE (1960) Proteins associated with the thyroid hormones. Physiol Rev 40: 415–489

Robbins J, Rall JE (1983) The iodine containing hormones. In: Gray CH, James VHT (eds) Hormones in blood, 3rd edn. Academic, London, pp 219–265

Robbins J, Cheng SY, Gershengorn MC, Glinoer D, Cahnmann HJ, Edelnoch H (1978) Thyroxine transport proteins of plasma. Molecular properties and biosynthesis. Recent Prog Horm Res 34: 477–517

Rosen HN, Benson MD, Liepnicks J et al (1991) Thyroxine interactions with transthyretin: a comparison of 10 different naturally occurring transthyretin variants. 10th International Thyroid Conference, February 3–8, The Hague

Ross HA, Exalto N, Kioppenborg PWC, Beuraad TJ (1989) Thyroid hormone binding in early pregnancy and the risk of spontaneous abortion. Eur J Obstet Gynecol Reprod Biol 32: 129–136

Rushebrook JI, Becker E, Schussler GC, Divino CM (1995) Identification of a human serum albumin species associated with familial dysalbuminemic hyperthyroxinemia. J Clin Endocrinol Metab 80: 461–467

Sapin R, Gasser F, Chambron J (1989) Hyperthyroxinemia familiale avec dysalbuminémie: dépistage sur 21 000 patients à l'occasion d'un bilan thyroïden. Pathol Biol (Paris) 37: 785–789

Sarne DH, Refetoff S, Nelson JC, Linarelli LG (1989) A new inherited abnormality of thyroxine-binding globulin (TBG-San Diego) with decreased affinity for thyroxine and triiodothyronine. J Clin Endocrinol Metab 68: 114–119

Scatchard G (1949) The attractions of proteins for small molecules and ions. Ann N Y Acad Sci 52: 660–672

Schreiber G, Aldred AR, Jaworowski A, Milsson C, Achen MG, Segal MB (1990) Thyroxine transport from blood to brain via transthyretin synthesis in choroid plexus. Am J Physiol 258: R338–R345

Schussler GC (1990) Thyroxine-binding proteins. Thyroid 1: 25–34

Sparre LS (1989) Maternal free thyroxine and thyroxine-binding globulin during pregnancy ending in congenital malformations in the offspring. Gynecol Obstet Invest 27: 19–21

Sterling K, Brenner MA (1966) Free thyroxine in human serum: simplified measurement with the aid of magnesium precipitation. J Clin Invest 45: 153–161

Sterling K, Hegedus A (1962) Measurement of free thyroxine concentration in human serum. J Clin Invest 41: 1031–1040

Stockigt JR, Dyer SA, Mohr VS, White EL, Barlow JW (1986) Specific methods to identify plasma binding abnormalities in euthyroid hyperthyroxinemia. J Clin Endocrinol Metab 62: 230–233

Stockigt JR (1983) Hyperthyroxinemia secondary to drugs and acute illness. Endocrinologist 1: 67–73

Stockigt JR, Topliss DJ, Barlow JW, White EL, Hurley DM, Taft P (1981) Familial euthyroid thyroxine excess: an appropriate response to abnormal throxine binding associated with albumin. J Clin Endocrinol Metab 53: 353–354

Stockigt JR, Stevens V, White EL, Barlow JW (1983) Unbound analog radioimmunoassays for free thyroxine measure the albumin-bound hormone fraction. Clin Chem 29: 1408–1410

Strunge P (1974) Familial thyroxine-binding globulin deficiency. A study of three Danish families. Acta Med Scand 195: 5–9

Sunthornthepvarakul T, Angkeow P, Weiss RE, Hayashi Y, Refetoff S (1994) A missense mutation in the albumin gene produces familial disalbuminemic hyperthyroxinemia in 8 unrelated families. Biochem Biophys Res Commun 202: 781–787

Sviridov OV, Ermolenko MN, Karpyza EI, Strel'chyonok OA (1991) Human thyroid hormone-binding IgM: isolation from human serum, binding properties and effects on thyroid hormone interaction with plasma membranes of human placenta. 73rd Annual Meeting of the American Endocrine Society, June 19–22, Washington

Takamatsu J, Ando M, Weinberg M, Refeoff S (1986) Isoelectric focusing of variant thyroxine-binding globulin in American blacks: increased heat lability and reduced serum concentration. J Clin Endocrinol Metab 63: 80–87

Takamatsu J, Ohsawa N (1990) Diagnosis of familial dysalbuminemic hyperthyroxinemia and investigation of the nature of the variant albumin. Bull Osaka Med Coll 36: 35–45

Takamatsu J, Refetoff S, Charbonneau M, Dussault J (1987) Two new inherited defects of the thyroxine-binding globulin (TBG) molecule presenting as partial TBG deficiency. J Clin Invest 79: 833–840

Takeda K, Mori Y, Sobieszczyk S, Seo H, Dick M, Watson F, Flink IL, Seino S, Bell G, Refetoff S (1989) Sequence of the variant thyroxine-binding globulin of Australian aborigines. J Clin Invest 83: 1344–1348

Tanaka S, Starr P (1959) An euthyroid man without thyroxine-binding globulin. J Clin Endocrinol 19: 485–486

Tragardh L, Anundi H, Rask L, Sege K, Peterson PA (1980) On the stoichiometry of the interaction between prealbumin and retinol-binding protein. J Biol Chem 255: 9243

Trent JM, Flink IL, Morkin E, Van Tuinen P, Ledbetter DH (1987) Localization of the human thyroxine-binding globuline gene to the long arm of the X-chromosome (Xq 21–22). Am J Hum Genet 41: 428–435

Van Jaarsveld PP, Edelhoch H, Goodman DS, Robbins J (1973) The interaction of human plasma retinol-binding protein with prealbumin. J Biol Chem 248: 4698

Wakonig P, Költringer P, Lind P, Eber O, Wawschinek O (1987) Methods for determining protein binding of thyroid hormones and T4- and T3-autoantibodies. Acta Med Austriaca 15: 15–19

Waltz MR, Pullma TN, Takeda K, Sobiexzczyk P, Refetoff S (1990) Molecular basis for the properties of the thyroxine-binding globulin-slow variant in American blacks. J Endocrinol Invest 13: 343–349

Wawschinek O, Leopold B, Aktuna D, Eber O, Lind P (1987) Radial immunodiffusion method in thyroid hormone autoantibody determination. Acta Med Austriaca 2: 37–40

Weiss RE, Sunthornthepvarakul T, Angkeow P, Marcus-Bagley D, Cox N, Alper CA, Refetoff S (1995) Linkage of familial dysalbuminemic hyperthyroxinemia to the albumin gene in a large Amish kindred. J Clin Endocrinol Metab 80: 116–121

Whitecar JP, Bodey GP, Harris JE, Freireich EJ (1970) Current concepts of L-asparaginase. N Engl J Med 282: 732

Wynne AG, Heufelder AE, Klee GG, Gharib H (1992) Familial dysalbuminemic hyperthyroxinemia: data on 29 consecutive patients. Thyroid 2(S): S18(A)

Yabu U, Amino N, Nakatari K, Ichihara K, Azukizawa M, Miyai K (1980) Graves' disease associated with elevated thyroxine-binding globulin concentrations. J Clin Endocrinol Metab 51: 325–329

Yabu Y, Amir SM, Ruiz M, Braverman LE, Ingbar SH (1985) Heterogeneity of thyroxine binding by serum albumins in normal subjects and patients with familial dysalbuminemic hyperthyroxinemia. J Clin Endocrinol Metab 60: 451–459

Yabu Y, Miyai K, Kobayashi A, Miki K, Doi K, Amatsu J, Mozai T, Matsuzuka F, Kuma K (1987) A new type of albumin with predominantly increased affinity for 3,3',5-triiodothyronine in a patient with Graves' disease. J Endocrinol Invest 10: 163–168
Yamamori I, Mori Y, Seo H, Hirooka Y, Imamura S, Miura Y, Matsui N, Oiso Y (1991) Nucleotide deletion resulting in frameshift as a possible cause of complete thyroxine-binding globulin deficiency in six Japanese families. J Clin Endocrinol Metab 73: 262–267
Yeo PPB, Yabu Y, Etzkorn JR, Rajatanavin R, Braverman LE, Ingbar SH (1987) A four generation study of familial dysalbuminemic hyperthyroxinemia: diagnosis in the presence of an acquired excess of thyroxine-binding globulin. J Endocrinol Invest 10: 33–38
Young RA, Stoffer SS, Braverman LE (1987) Familial dysalbuminemic hyperthyroxinemia associated with a primary thyroid disease. Am J Med 82: 221–223

Subject Index

Index of Volumes 88–90 Current Topics in Pathology

D. HARMS, Alveolar Rhabdomyosarcoma: A Prognostically Unfavorable Rhabdomyosarcoma Type and Its Necessary Distinction from Embryonal Rhabdomyosarcoma

D. SCHMIDT, Malignant Peripheral Neuroectodermal Tumor

A.O. CAVAZZANA, V. NINFO, R. TIRABOSCO, A. MONTALDI, and R. FRUNZIO, Leiomyosarcoma

C.D.M. FLETCHER, Malignant Peripheral Nerve Sheath Tumors

C.D.M. FLETCHER, Rare Soft Tissue Sarcomas

Volume 90: Oral Pathology. Edited by G. SEIFERT

D.M. WILLIAMS, Mucocutaneous Conditions Affecting the Mouth

C. SCULLY, New Aspects of Oral Viral Diseases

P.A. REICHART, Oral Pathology of Acquired Immunodeficiency Syndrome and Oro-facial Kaposi's Sarcoma

R.C.K. JORDAN and P.M. SPEIGHT, Extranodal Non-Hodgkin's Lymphomas of the Oral Cavity

K.A.A.S. WARNAKULASURIYA and N.W. JOHNSON, Importance of Proliferation Markers in Oral Pathology

P.J. SLOOTWEG, Suppressor Protein p53 and Its Occurrence in Oral Tumours

A.G.M. SCHOLES and J.K. FIELD, Genomic Instability in Head and Neck Cancer

A. BURKHARDT, Oncogenes and Growth Factor Receptors as Diagnostic and Prognostic Markers in Precancers and Cancers of the Oral Mucosa

SPRINGER NATURE

GPSR Compliance

The European Union's (EU) General Product Safety Regulation (GPSR) is a set of rules that requires consumer products to be safe and our obligations to ensure this.

If you have any concerns about our products, you can contact us on ProductSafety@springernature.com

In case Publisher is established outside the EU, the EU authorized representative is:

Springer Nature Customer Service Center GmbH
Europaplatz 3
69115 Heidelberg, Germany

FSC
www.fsc.org
MIX
Papier | Fördert gute Waldnutzung
FSC® C083411

Kolibri 360 GmbH
Ferdinand-Jühlke-Straße 7
99095 Erfurt, Deutschland
produktsicherheit@kolibri360.de